running**FIT**

in association with

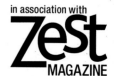

ZeSt
MAGAZINE

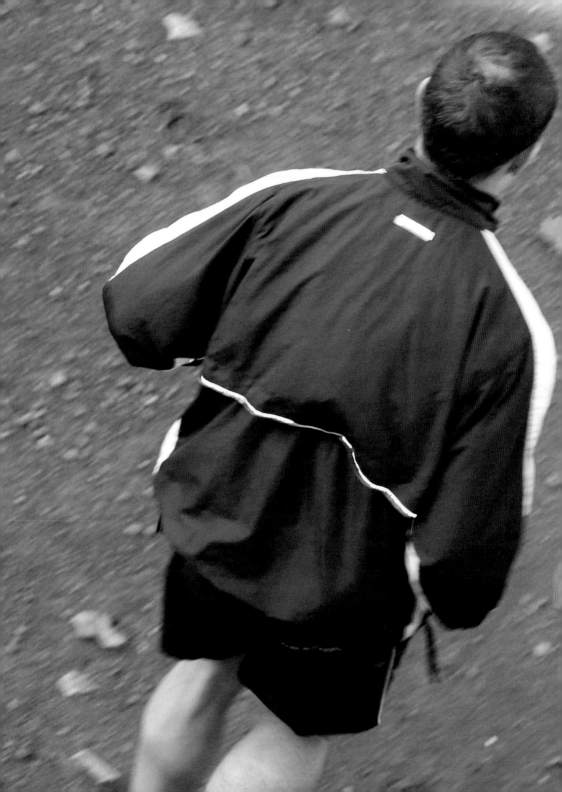

running**FIT**

Jamie Baird

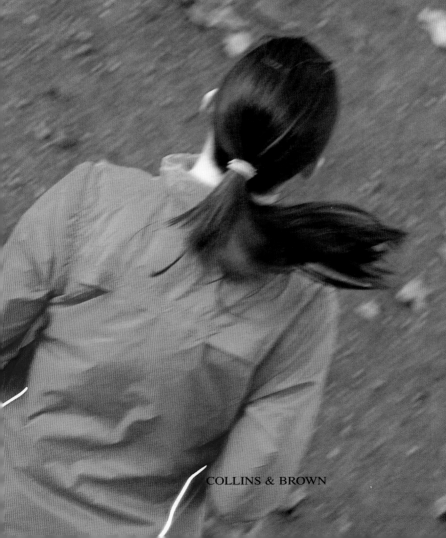

COLLINS & BROWN

First published in Great Britain in 2006 by
Collins & Brown
The Chrysalis Building
Bramley Road
London W10 6SP

An imprint of Anova Books Company Ltd

Distributed in the United States and Canada by
Sterling Publishing Co, 387 Park Avenue South, New York, NY 10016, USA.

The National Magazine Company Ltd.
Zest is the registered trademark of The National Magazine Company Ltd

1 3 5 7 9 8 6 4 2

British Library Cataloguing-in-Publication Data:
A catalogue record for this book is available from the British Library.

ISBN 1 84340 332 3

Commissioning Editor: Victoria Alers-Hankey
Design Manager: Gemma Wilson
Editors: Emma Dickens and Jane Ellis
Photographs: pages 2-35, 41, 52-61, 68, 94-121 Guy Hearn, pages 64-67, 71-93 Micheal Wicks
Senior Production Controller: Morna McPherson
Designer: Simon Daley
Model: Jade Cresswell

Reproduction by Anorax Ltd
Printed and bound in China

Acknowledgements
A huge special thanks to Emilie Hartigan for her awesome journalistic skills, who has always been
there and slaved away tirelessly in Geneva putting my garbled text into readable English. To my
Mum and Dad for their encouragement over the years and consistent support in all my projects
and sporting life. To Anne Kibel at TFA and Victoria Alers-Hankey at Collins & Brown for all of
their help. To my clients for helping me hone my skills and allowing me to be part of their lives.
And lastly to the Ganoush, one day I might get you into a pair of runners.

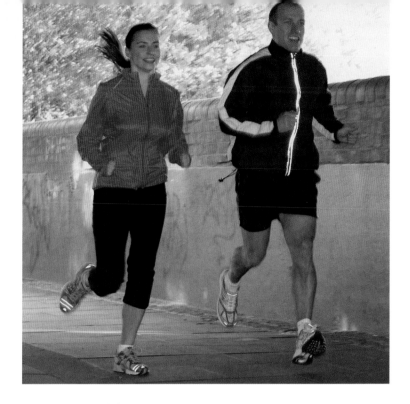

Contents

Introduction

I have been running even since I can remember. Even as a kid, I was obsessed. I ran morning, noon and night. I recall waking up early to run before school – putting in a quick 3–4 miles and then logging more miles during track practice in the evenings. By age 12, I'd run my first half

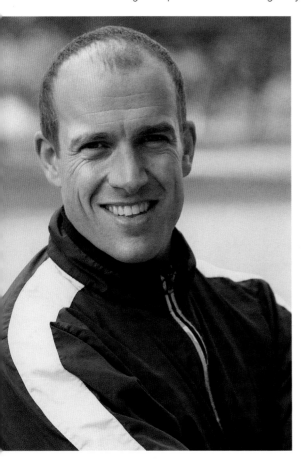

marathon, and my second came at age 13. Looking back now, I know that I was far too young to be running on the roads, but we didn't know then what we know today. During those pre-teen years, I was probably running up to 30 miles per week, but I loved every step.

My third half marathon, an attempt to break 1hr 25 mins, ended in tears and was followed by numerous visits to the physio for regular treatments. In fact, I think I was one of the only boys who was allowed to turn up late to school because he had to go the Leicester Royal for his physio treatment. The physio, thank God, saved me from having to undergo surgery. He gave me exercises to do in the mornings before school and, again, in the evenings. It wasn't fun, but it did the trick. Today, I run on roads without a problem and, (touch wood!),

I have never needed surgery. Despite my luck, sheer determination, drive and love of running it nearly ruined my knees well and truly. I was lucky enough to have people around me who gave great advice and could offer simple treatment options. However, what really saved me in the end was my willingness to listen to them and take their advice.

At my athletics club I was a jack of all trades and master of none. I was the one who would compete in events just to earn the club a few more valuable points. The hurdles became a no-no when they became taller than me.

I am still making efforts to improve my running today. I don't do it because I have to; I do it because I can. I even enjoy running in the rain or the snow but I am not so keen on the wind. For me it's an escape, bringing back a lot of great memories.

As a fitness trainer, I run with many of my clients. I enjoy the outdoors, the fresh air. In fact, I think that the last time I ran properly on a treadmill was some 12 years ago. Rain or shine, I am always ready for a good run, though my clients aren't necessarily thrilled by my enthusiasm. Luckily for me, my clients have a wide range of fitness abilities, so I have the chance to train at different intensities and keep it interesting. After all, whether jogging in the park or pushing through the last 2 miles of a marathon, there is a style of running to accommodate every taste – you just need to find the right mix for you!

This book will provide you with all the basics you need to build an enjoyable and effective running programme. The first few chapters will lay the framework, explaining important physiological and practical information that will inform your specific programme choices. We will review such important areas as safety, injury prevention and nutrition. I strongly recommend you take the time to carefully read these early chapters before moving onto the second half of the book. Good training decisions are the result of proper understanding, so you need a comprehensive understanding of these fundamentals before getting started.

However, this is only a book, and at the end of the day, any real results will be decided by your motivation, commitment and, well, sheer determination. Put your head into training along with your body and you will see improvements. But most importantly, don't be afraid of the hard work; after all, anything worth having requires a real effort!

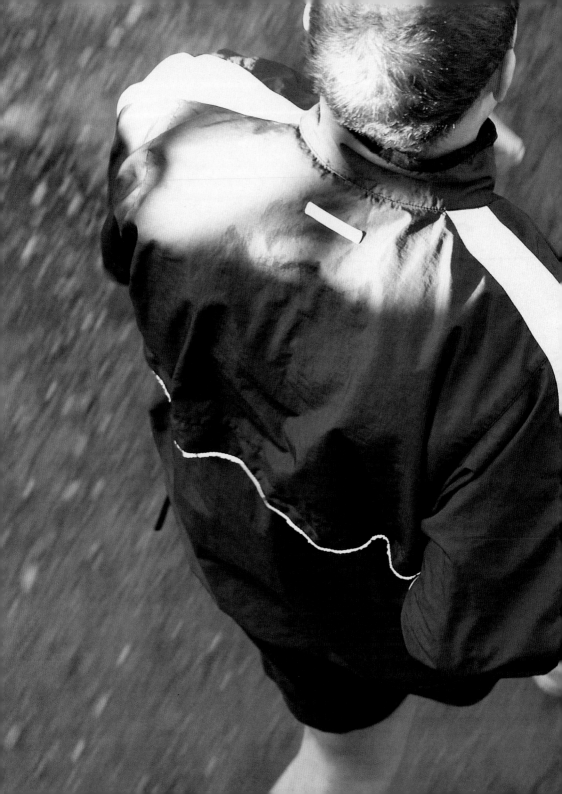

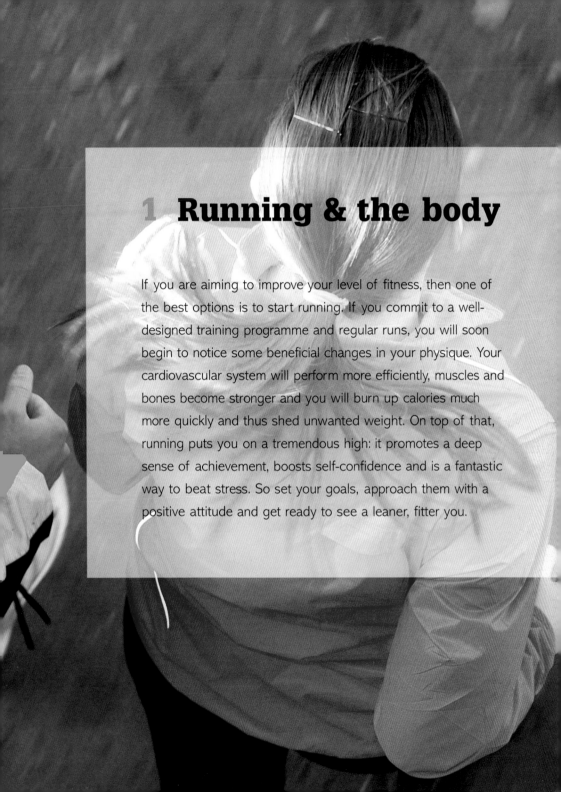

1 Running & the body

If you are aiming to improve your level of fitness, then one of the best options is to start running. If you commit to a well-designed training programme and regular runs, you will soon begin to notice some beneficial changes in your physique. Your cardiovascular system will perform more efficiently, muscles and bones become stronger and you will burn up calories much more quickly and thus shed unwanted weight. On top of that, running puts you on a tremendous high: it promotes a deep sense of achievement, boosts self-confidence and is a fantastic way to beat stress. So set your goals, approach them with a positive attitude and get ready to see a leaner, fitter you.

Choosing fitness

If you are reading this book, the chances are you're not entirely satisfied with your current level of fitness, but there's no need to feel embarrassed about it. You're in good company, as the profitability of today's weight-loss industry proves. In the quest for a perfect waistline, many of us have tried a fad diet or spent loads on muscle-building supplements – but the sad fact is that 'get fit quick' products don't work. After all, if fitness came in a can, wouldn't it have caught on by now?

Real fitness, the sort that affects your entire physiology, builds your self-confidence and improves your quality of life, requires good, old-fashioned sweat. This may not be what you want to hear, but it is the truth. If you want to be fit, you need to be focused. You need to be willing to invest the time and energy to meet your goals. You need to be ready to push through moments of laziness; to accept that there will be trying times when every ounce of motivation is lacking.

You need to look at the process of building fitness and health as a journey, an ongoing process that changes with each passing year. The task of getting fit at 25 is quite different from getting fit at 30 or 50. But no matter your age, there is no reason not to take the plunge. The benefits of a well-designed exercise programme will begin to affect your body positively from day one, regardless of your previous fitness level and age. It is nature's way of motivating us to keep at it.

Running is one of a variety of ways to build a fitter body. Other options include cycling, aerobics, rowing, weightlifting, team sports ... the list is endless. But running is the ideal core activity for any fitness plan – allowing you to build a base of cardiovascular fitness and achieve your healthiest weight naturally.

So why run?

Running produces numerous changes throughout the body, many of which are necessary for adaptation and improvement. Regular running or cardiovascular exercise strengthens the heart and helps to create a better oxygen transportation system. It generates an increase in capillaries (which supply the muscles with nutrients), mitochondria (the powerhouses in the muscle) and red blood cells (which carry the oxygen to the muscles). All these improvements lead to an elevated oxygen uptake and better health.

The hardest thing about running is getting out of the door. It is moving past that 'throw in the towel' moment, that critical point between thinking about doing it and actually going to get changed. As soon as you slip into those workout clothes that's it, you're going running. What you need is that extra bit of motivational information to get you lacing up those shoes. Let's start with the obvious benefits:

- ▶ Great way to burn loads of calories.
- ▶ Weight loss.
- ▶ Healthier lifestyle.
- ▶ Strengthens the heart and lungs.
- ▶ To increase current fitness levels (or lack of).
- ▶ Strengthens bones, joints, ligaments, tendons and muscles.
- ▶ Because you can.
- ▶ Reduces the signs of ageing.
- ▶ It could help you live longer.

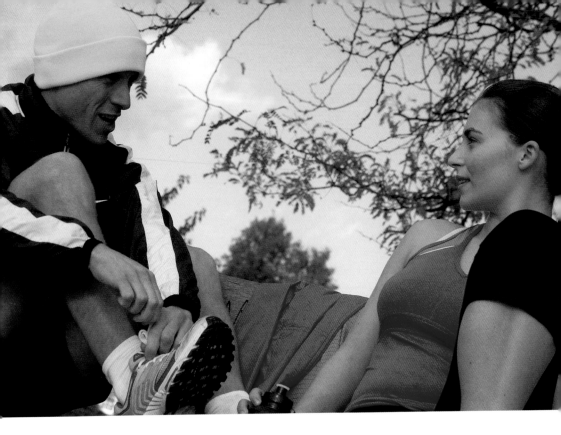

And the benefits of running extend beyond the physical:

- ▶ A sense of freedom.
- ▶ A happier, leaner, smarter self.
- ▶ Better sleep.
- ▶ Better stress management.
- ▶ Increased confidence, elevated self-esteem.
- ▶ A deep sense of satisfaction and achievement.

And before I forget one of its top selling points – running is FREE. You don't need a fancy gym, the latest high-tech equipment or a professional trainer. In fact, when it comes to running, almost anyone, anywhere, at any time can participate. If you are looking for a low cost workout, nothing beats running. All you need is a good pair of trainers.

The chemistry of conditioning

If all that hasn't convinced you, then maybe a more in-depth review of the physiological benefits of running will do the trick:

Blood pressure

Blood pressure is the stress exerted on the arterial walls with each heartbeat. A blood pressure reading is expressed by two figures (120/80 mm/hg). The upper figure is the systolic reading, and is the peak pressure produced by each heartbeat; the lower figure, the diastolic pressure, is a measure of the level to which the pressure falls before the next heartbeat.

An elevated blood pressure increases one's risk of CHD (Coronary Heart Disease), by putting extra strain on the walls of the arteries. There are many contributing factors to elevated blood pressure, including being overweight, poor diet, high salt intake, too much alcohol, stress and not enough exercise. Running is one of the most effective ways to improve your blood pressure over time.

Healthy heart

Your resting heart rate (RHR) is the lowest number of times per minute that your heart beats. For the majority of people, it should fall below 70 beats per minute (bpm).

When you train and improve your fitness, your body becomes more efficient at delivering oxygen to the muscles. As a result, your resting heart rate naturally lowers. Just 8–16 km (5–10 miles) of running per week – that's only 1.5–2.5 km (1–1.5 miles) 4–6 times a week – can reduce the risk of a heart attack by 20 per cent.

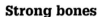

Strong bones

Running is a great way, along with other weight-bearing activities, to help increase or maintain the density of your bones. This is particularly relevant to women, who lose bone density with age, making them more susceptible to debilitating conditions like osteoporosis and osteoarthritis.

Body weight

Being overweight puts unnecessary strain on the body's functions. The more calories you put in and the fewer you burn, the more you will store. Running is a great way to burn additional calories and achieve a negative net calorific balance. When you combine running or other exercise with healthy balanced nutrition, you should see a drop in your weight.

Metabolic rate

When it comes to weight loss, most people these days are familiar with the importance of metabolism. Your resting metabolic rate is the number of calories your body burns in a state of inactivity. If weight loss is a priority for you, it is useful to find ways to boost this base rate. There are many ways to increase your metabolic rate, however the most effective is through weight training and/or lifting weights. The more muscle you have the more calories you will burn on a daily basis.

Cholesterol

The two main forms of cholesterol are Low Density Lipoprotein (LDL) and High Density Protein (HDL). Your body needs cholesterol to function; however, if too much LDL gets laid down in the walls of the arteries it will cause them to harden and narrow. The HDL cholesterol is good cholesterol, which strips LDL from the artery walls. Vigorous aerobic exercise, such as running, reduces LDL and raises HDL.

Different approaches for different aims

There are a number of different reasons to incorporate running into your exercise regimen. But perhaps you have a specific training focus, and are wondering how best to tailor your programme to meet your personal requirements? Running for weight loss requires a different approach from running to improve speed or competitive success. While you can lose excess weight through any running training, the real key to long-term weight loss and maintenance is a sustainable exercise/nutritional programme – you needn't worry about breaking the land speed record your first year out. In fact, if you are beginning with a lowered level of fitness, trying to train as a sprinter is counter-productive and even dangerous. The key is to determine your priorities at the outset and build your programme to suit.

So how is running for weight loss different from running for speed improvements or cardiovascular conditioning? It's all to do with the different activity zones that the body experiences during exercise. All human movement requires energy. The intensity and duration of an activity determines which method of energy production the body will use.

Activities that demand sudden bursts of energy – such as running up a steep hill – require a large and immediate production; endurance activities – like running long distances – require energy to be produced more slowly and consistently over a longer period of time.

Depending on the intensity and duration of an activity – as well as your fitness level – the body will utilise energy from different sources: the Aerobic System (long-term energy) and, the Anaerobic (short-term and immediate energy) System.

The use of oxygen by the body's cells is known as oxygen uptake or consumption. At rest, the body consumes approximately 3.5 ml of oxygen per kg of bodyweight per minute (ml/kg/min). The maximum amount of oxygen a person can consume (via the lungs), transport (via the heart and arteries)

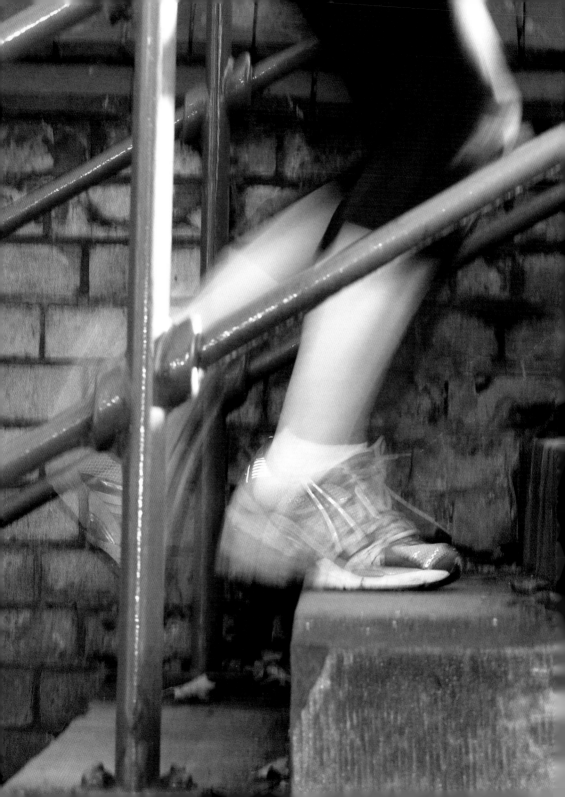

and use (via the muscles) provides enough information to determine an individual's fitness level. The more oxygen consumed, transported and used; the higher the achievable exercise intensity and, consequently, the fitter the person will be. When we train, our bodies adapt in order to utilise more oxygen. Some of the adaptations made are:

▶ An increase in the number of red blood cells (which carry the oxygen to the working muscles).
▶ Increased efficiency of the lungs (more oxygen passes into the bloodstream and carbon dioxide is expelled).
▶ A greater number of capillaries within the muscle (which allows for better distribution of oxygen within the muscle).
▶ A greater number and increased size of mitochondria (where the energy is created) within the muscle.

All these changes combine to create a healthier and fitter system. Cardiovascular function improves; circulation is more efficient; excess weight dissolves and lung capacity (pulmonary health) improves. This is why consistent participation in an exercise programme can lower one's risk of fatal health risks such as a stroke and coronary artery disease.

The Aerobic System – long-term energy

The Aerobic System is the most important energy system. Our bodies rely on it constantly for normal functioning in everyday life. It produces energy in the presence of oxygen. As the intensity of an exercise increases, the exercising muscles use increasing amounts of oxygen, causing the Aerobic System to burn more fuel. Because aerobic energy production utilises carbohydrates and fats as fuel, maintaining an active Aerobic System is often cited as the key element in healthy weight management. A person's aerobic capacity is determined by the efficiency of the cardiovascular system in carrying oxygen to the muscles. Cardiovascular fitness is measured in terms of aerobic capacity or Max VO2. To increase aerobic fitness the heart rate needs to be elevated (120+ bpm) for a period of 20–30+ minutes as often as possible.

The Anaerobic System – short-term energy

The Anaerobic System is the body's way of producing energy without having to depend on oxygen. The body switches into anaerobic mode when the intensity of exercise increases to a point where the heart and lungs can't supply enough oxygen to meet the body's energy demands. Instead, the Anaerobic System uses specialised chemicals reserved in the body to provide the necessary energy. These chemicals are in limited supply, meaning the body can only work anaerobically for brief periods. To develop your cardiovascular system totally, both Aerobic and Anaerobic Systems must be trained.

At rest, your muscles are working aerobically. As exercise intensity increases from rest to gentle jogging to sprinting, the body's demand for oxygen also increases. At higher intensities it becomes more of a challenge for your cardiovascular system to deliver enough oxygen to the working muscles. If muscle cells are not trained to function under the additional stress of exercise, they may not be able to extract the available oxygen from the blood as intensity increases. Consequently, the delivery and utilisation of oxygen to the exercising muscles will be inadequate. At this point, your muscles have to shift to the Anaerobic System to be able to continue exercising. When shifting to anaerobic mode, your body will make use of two different components depending on the situational needs:

▶ **Immediate energy** Provides instantaneous energy to react immediately to a given situation, such as a short sprint, catching a bus or responding to danger. Very short duration: 1–10 seconds of energy.
▶ **Short-term energy** Responsible for providing the energy needed to make it to the top of a steep hill or sprint to the finishing line. Short duration: 60–180 seconds of energy.

At any given time, all three energy systems (aerobic, immediate anaerobic and short-term anaerobic) are functioning simultaneously; the intensity, the duration of the exercise and your fitness level determine what percentage of each system is being used.

Determining your training zone

Now that you have the basics on how energy systems work, it is time to consider the best way to train for your specific goals. The easiest way to control your exercise programme – maintaining intensity and tracking improvements – is by monitoring your heart rate (HR). Obviously, as we move from aerobic to anaerobic levels of activity, our heart rate increases to accommodate the body's needs for energy. By tracking our pulse, it is possible to ensure we are training at the right level – neither too much nor too little.

The simplest way to do this is with an HR monitor (see page 31). If you're new to CV training, an HR monitor consists of a wristwatch and a transmitter worn around the chest. The transmitter picks up the signals of your heart, sending them to the watch. It's that simple: no wires, no stopping to take your pulse, no complicated arithmetic. It allows you to customise any fitness programme, tailoring the type of workout to suit target HR zones and specific goals. Essentially, it keeps you working effectively.

Calculating your heart-rate zones

So how do you find exactly which zone you are in at any given time? The first step in planning your training programme is calculating your personal zones, based on your resting heart rate (RHR). Once you have determined what your base rate is, then you can easily compute which pulse corresponds with which zone.

The table on the opposite page will guide you through the various calculations necessary for determining your resting, working and maximum heart rate.

Putting it into Practice

I know that all of these equations can be intimidating at the start. The bottom line is that running will improve your fitness, regardless of what the numbers say. However, knowing your different HR zones can only help to improve your fitness level over time. By calculating your personal ranges, you will have all the information you need to exercise with maximum efficiency and minimum risk.

By combining your HR training with well-designed training plans, you will achieve your goals. Below is a listing of the various HR zones:

The Zones

Aerobic Zone (AZ)

▶ Roughly 60–75 per cent of (Working Heart Rate) WHR .
▶ The easiest zone to sustain for extended periods.
▶ Fat loss and foundation building zone.
▶ Beginners need 4–8 weeks of conditioning to build fitness before working beyond AZ.

Lactate Threshold Zone (LTZ)

▶ 80–90 per cent of WHR.
▶ Interval training: Alternate between LTZ and AZ, spending 5–10 minutes in each. Repeat cycle three times. Intervals help your body acclimatise to increased lactate build-up.

Max VO2 Zone (MVZ)

▶ 90–100 per cent of WHR.
▶ Once-a-week intervals improve strength and power.
▶ Interval training: Warm up in AZ for 10 minutes; do 3–10 cycles of 1–3 minutes at MVZ, alternating equal time recovery; follow with a 10–20 minute AZ cool-down.

How to calculate your training heart rates

To measure your Resting Heart Rate (RHR)

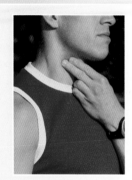

► Make sure that you are in a relaxed state. The most accurate way to correctly measure your RHR is to take your pulse after a good night's sleep.
► Locate your pulse (either at your wrist or at your neck).
► Count for 60 seconds.

Example: Mr X: 60bpm (15 beats in a 15-second interval multiplied by 4). bpm = beats per minute

To estimate your Maximum Heart Rate (MHR)
Method 1
For years the formula 220 − age was the standard method but this equation has several limiting factors. The formula can be inaccurate for up to + or − 10–15 beats. That said, it can provide a useful starting point.
Method 2
A slightly more accurate, though still imperfect, equation varies for men and women.
► Men: 214 − (0.8 x age)   ► Women: 209 − (0.9 x age)
Despite accounting for sex, this is still a one-size-fits-all approach and quite inaccurate for a great percentage of the population.
Method 3
To accurately measure your Maximum Heart Rate:
► Warm up for about 5 minutes and stretch if necessary.
► Once you are limber, run fast for 3 minutes, following with a recovery jog of 2–3 minutes.
► Repeat the hard 3-minute run, keeping an eye on your heart rate.
► Make a note of the highest value you achieve.

To measure your Working Heart Rate (WHR)
► Subtract your Resting Heart Rate from your Maximum Heart Rate.
Example: 186 bpm − 60 bpm = 126 bpm

How to work out your training zone

There are three broad training zones:
- ▶ 60–75 per cent – easy, long, slow distance.
- ▶ 80–90 per cent – moderate.
- ▶ 90–100 per cent – hard, to really push your fitness to new levels.

Find your training zone in five easy steps:
1. Find your Resting Heart Rate (see previous page).
2. Find your Maximum Heart Rate (see previous page).
3. Find your Working Heart Rate (see previous page).
4. Multiply your WHR by your desired training zone percentage.
5. Take that figure and add it to your Resting Heart Rate. The final figure is your personal target heart rate.

Training Heart Rates for Mr X
126 (WHR) x 60 per cent = 75 + 60 (RHR) = 135bpm
126 (WHR) x 75 per cent = 94 + 60 (RHR) = 154bpm
126 (WHR) x 85 per cent = 107 + 60 (RHR) = 167bpm
126 (WHR) x 95 per cent = 120 + 60 (RHR) = 180bpm

Note to Beginners
If you are new to exercise, you might find your resting heart rate on the higher than average side. As your fitness levels improve, this will adjust, so re-take your resting pulse every 2–4 weeks in order to adjust your working heart rate.

Running for your heart and head

An often overlooked benefit of exercise is its positive impact on one's mental health, emotional stability and general sense of wellbeing. Running is a particularly effective way of improving these. When you run, your body releases endorphins, the feel-good hormones that promote relaxation and alleviate depression. Over time, the chemical changes affected by the consistent release of endorphins will be obvious in all aspects of your daily life. Stress levels will be reduced and, consequently, challenges at work and at home will seem less daunting. Your confidence will improve, regardless of aesthetic changes, and you will feel generally more capable.

Because running is a challenge, you really do have to learn to motivate yourself to participate: Positive Mental Attitude is essential. If you don't think you can improve, then the chances are you won't. By building this PMA outlook, you will actually be changing negative thought patterns that might be sabotaging other aspects of your life.

The bottom line – taking responsibility

By maintaining a proper balance of all aspects of training – whether by observing the necessary rest days or pushing yourself to maintain effective intensity during a run – you will meet your goals. The most important thing to remember is that exercising the body is all in the mind. It sounds contradictory, but the truth is that if you want to make improvements to your physical health, you need to learn how to train your head. Our behaviour dictates our health – so if you are feeling a bit the worse for wear, it is time to re-evaluate your lifestyle and make proactive changes.

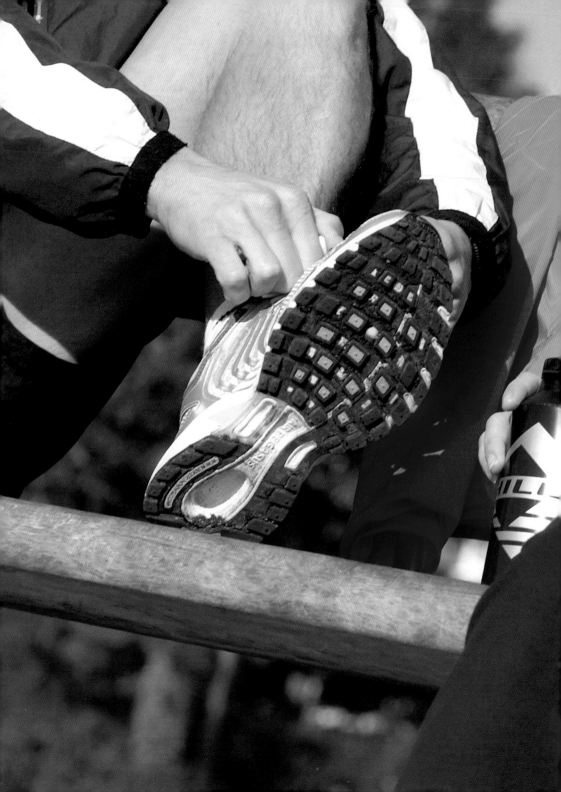

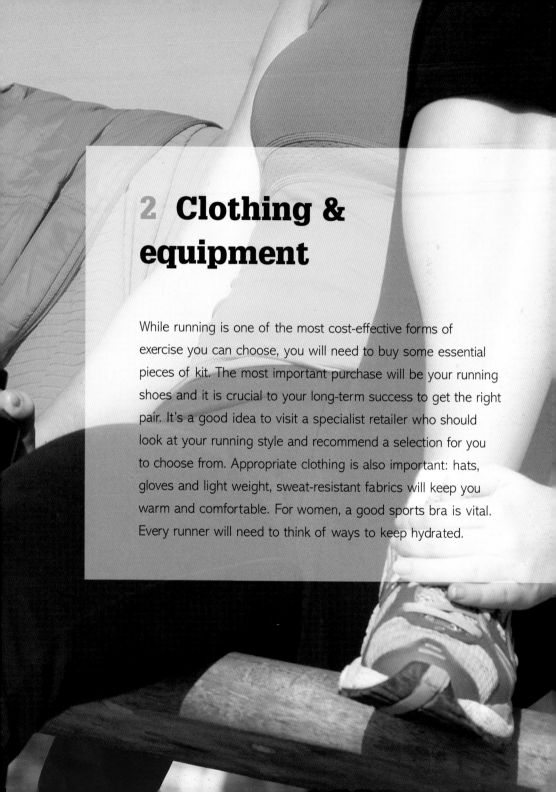

2 Clothing & equipment

While running is one of the most cost-effective forms of exercise you can choose, you will need to buy some essential pieces of kit. The most important purchase will be your running shoes and it is crucial to your long-term success to get the right pair. It's a good idea to visit a specialist retailer who should look at your running style and recommend a selection for you to choose from. Appropriate clothing is also important: hats, gloves and light weight, sweat-resistant fabrics will keep you warm and comfortable. For women, a good sports bra is vital. Every runner will need to think of ways to keep hydrated.

Proper gear

Shoes

Your shoes will be the most expensive part of your running kit. They will also be the piece you most regularly replace. So how do you select the right pair? And how long will they last? The answers to these questions depend on the quality of the shoes and how often they are used.

Shoe wear-and-tear is the result of many individual factors, such as their treatment, what weekly mileage they're doing, their original quality, your bodyweight, the chosen terrain, and, of course, your running style.

Choosing your shoes

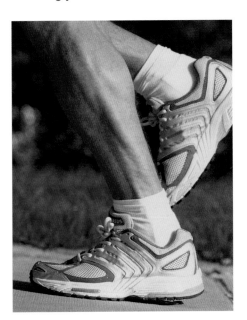

Buying any pair of shoes is hard, but buying a pair of running shoes can be even more difficult, with endless ranges, makes, models and prices – not to mention the problem of finding the right fit for your foot and running style. Keep in mind the fact that a top-of-the-range shoe is not going to make you run faster! It might even be inappropriate for your foot and do more harm than good – so you need good advice.

Your feet in motion

When you run or walk, your feet tend to roll inwards. This is known as pronation. However, some people's feet roll inwards more than others, which over time can put added stress on the shins, ankles, knees, hips and lower back.

Motion control shoes counteract this movement by having harder, more supportive foam in the mid-sole, which slows down the pronating motion. Some runners have perfect gaits and need little control, while others who have only a slight inwards roll can make do with a stability shoe.

▶ **The neutral foot** The runner has a neutral gait, the foot stays properly aligned when it impacts with the ground, keeping the rest of the body in line.

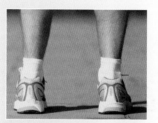

▶ **The Overpronator:** On impact with the ground the foot/ankle rolls inwards. The knock-on effect can lead to a whole host of injuries from the Achilles tendon upwards.

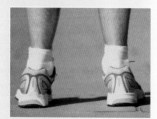

▶ **The Underpronator (supination):** On impact with the ground, the foot does not roll in enough to accommodate the motion. Over time, this can put stress on the lower back and hip region.

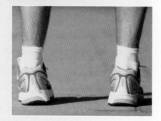

As you run, you absorb 1½–3 times your weight throughout your body. So you can see why the right shoe is essential. In fact, choosing the right shoe is probably the most important thing you can do before you embark on a running programme. Check the underside of an old pair of running shoes or even a pair of flat shoes and see where the most wear-and-tear appears on the outsole. This will help you assess your style of motion.

Entry-level running shoes are a great choice for first timers. However, they might prove insufficient and cause injury if you need a more substantial shoe due to excessive pronation or impact forces. If the shoe does not feel right, then it probably isn't. Comfort is a great indication of how suitable the shoe is. Remember, if you are wearing the wrong shoe for your foot type you can end up in all sorts of difficulties.

The best strategy is to visit a specialist retailer. This should take a lot of the weight off your shoulders. They can explain all the technological jargon and watch how you run, and you can ask specific questions, which in turn will help them choose a suitable selection of shoes for you.

A moderately priced pair of trainers is normally sufficient for the majority of runners. Any shop that does not show you a range of shoes at different prices is not worth stepping into. Be aware of buying your shoes off the Internet, unless it's a model you've already had. With a little bit of research through the relevant running magazines you will find out who the real specialists are. A good specialist retailer will:

▶ Explain his chosen selection of shoes for you.
▶ Not just show you the most expensive shoe.
▶ Look at or ask about your running style.
▶ Look at your existing trainers to assess your form.
▶ Allow you to jog in them either outside or inside the shop.
▶ Possibly even film you running or scan your foot to get a more detailed look at your running style.

Types of shoes
- ► **Motion control shoes** These shoes are the most rigid and prevent the excessive inward roll associated with overpronation. They tend to be heavier but are extremely durable, so they are favoured by heavier/larger runners.
- ► **Cushioned shoes** These have the least support – they are ideal for a neutral runner.
- ► **Stability shoes** These provide good shock absorption, durability and medial support via a dual density mid-sole.
- ► **Off-road shoes** These tend to have a lot more lateral support and better outsoles for more grip and durability. Their construction is a lot more aggressive – some models are even waterproof.

Women's shoes

Women differ from men biomechanically in several respects, including their hip ratio. This means that a woman's hips are wider than a man's. It also means that the angle from a woman's hips to her knees is greater than the corresponding angle on a man. This biomechanical difference can cause women to strike the ground more on the outside of their foot. So when buying shoes, women should be particularly careful to receive proper advice on the best models and makes for their running style. It is a good idea for women who believe that they may have this tendency to take their used shoes with them when purchasing their next pair.

Quick buying tips

Your feet are largest at the end of the day, so buy your trainers in the afternoon or evening. Make sure that when you try them on you are able to wiggle your toes and the trainers don't constrict your foot width. Every running shoe will be slightly different, so your purchase should not be rushed and you should try on a selection before making your choice.

The weakest part of the shoe is the mid-sole, which gives the shoe its cushioning and absorbs much of your weight. Over time, this cushioning breaks down. On average, a well-made pair of running shoes will last for about 800 km (500 miles). But how you care for your shoes will have a great impact on how long they last. They will live longer if you only wear them for your workouts. In the event of them getting wet, you should be sure to dry them thoroughly before the next run. Remember to change your shoes every 500–800 km (300–500 miles). This does not mean you have to throw them away, just use them for something other than running.

Socks

Wearing socks also absorbs sweat from you feet and keeps your shoes from disintegrating and becoming smelly. Seamless socks are not essential but when running longer distances they are advisable.

Clothing

When running, the body generates heat, which you want to retain when running in cold temperatures. A good base layer will help you retain some of this warmth. You will need a lightweight material that draws sweat/moisture away from the skin. It is also good to remember that several layers of sweat resistant fabric are more effective for retaining heat than a single heavy garment. Ask your local sportswear retailer about their favourite brands.

Additional clothing accessories

► **Hat** Essential for cold weather days, a hat keeps you from losing up to 30 per cent of your body heat.

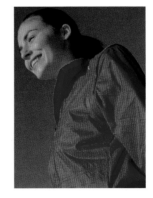

► **Gloves** Running gloves are thinner than the standard sets and most are specifically designed to wick the moisture away from your skin, keeping your hands warmer than normal, thicker models.

► **Gilets** Sleeveless outer garments worn over your base layer provide extra warmth while leaving your arms free.

Women's clothing

A sports bra is probably one of the most important pieces of kit every female runner can own. The fit should be snug, but not overly snug. A tight bra might chafe and prolonged wear of a badly sized bra can impede your circulation and hence your performance. Sports bras come in different styles and cuts – it is a matter of personal preference.

Training tools

Heart Rate (HR) Monitor HR monitors come in handy for tracking progress. They come in a variety of makes and models – test before you buy.
Stopwatch As the training schedules in Chapter 6 of this book are based around running for time, a stopwatch is an essential piece of kit. Relying on your dress watch is not going to be sufficient when you start having to record accurate times for specific runs. You can find a good selection of stopwatches at most sports shops and watch retailers. When looking to buy, make sure that you can read the numbers easily on the display and that the watch has an easy-to-use stopwatch function.

As you get into your running and start to experiment with intervals and speed work, you will need to look for a watch that includes lap, memory and countdown timer options.

Hydration options Staying hydrated is absolutely essential during training. If you are running for over 30 minutes, you will want to consider investing in one of the many types of water carrier on the market, such as a special water bottle carrying belt that snaps around your waist. I would advise against carrying water bottles in your hands as this can place stress on the shoulder joints and may lead to injury.

Wristbands for money If you are going out for a long run it is a good idea to carry some change, especially if you are not carrying any water. This way you can grab a quick drink. Many sports retailers carry wristbands with special compartments for change. They tend to double as reflective straps, so have a duel purpose.

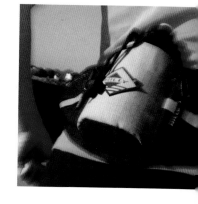

Weather – running in the elements

Running in bad weather is character building. Being out in the elements can re-energise you and increase your sense of accomplishment and satisfaction. That said though, getting outside for your workout is a great way to accelerate your fitness development, running in the elements can be a challenge, and the wrong gear can make it near impossible. But with the right clothing and a well-planned route, weather ceases to become the issue – in fact, you might even start to like the extra challenge. So go on, put on the gear and get outside – unless of course you're one of those fair-weather runners, only committed to running on treadmills or in the summer sunshine.

Rain

Rain can really ruin a great run. Just the idea of heavy, wet clothes, hair matted against your face and the uncomfortable possibility of being caught in a torrential downpour can send even the most committed runner back to their couch. In short, rain can kill a run before you even get out of the door! So what to do when the clouds set in? Invest in a high-visibility, top-quality waterproof jacket and you'll never know you've been out in the rain.

How to select proper rain gear
A good rain jacket has to be breathable. This means it needs to let the moisture out while keeping the rain from getting in. Most running gear retailers will be able to guide you towards the most effective products.

A final word on rainy day running
Just remember it's only water and you will only get wet!

Staying comfortable during cold weather

▶ Wear a microfibre shirt next to your skin. This will wick sweat away from the body.
▶ Wear a pair of gloves and a hat to cover your head and ears. Remember that you lose a large percentage of your body heat through your head.

Cold weather

Running in colder climates requires a few adaptations. Namely, you will need to spend more time warming up, and will have to equip yourself properly to avoid becoming chilled once the sweating starts. Sweating is not a great thing in cold temperatures, as the chilled sweat will increase body heat loss, so opting for quick-dry fabrics can be the key to a warm run.

Hot weather

Running in cold weather may be uncomfortable, but running in hot weather can be dangerous. Still, by taking a few simple precautions you can enjoy a run on the hottest of days. Dehydration is one of the most prevalent problems that runners encounter, and is particularly tricky for novices as in its early stages dehydration can be almost impossible to detect. By the time you feel thirsty, you are already very dehydrated. The best preventive measure is to carry a water bottle or wear a hydration pack. Running at cooler times of the day – morning and evening – can also cut down on potential danger.

The sun is another important consideration on hot days. Wearing a visor/cap, lightweight clothing and adequate sunscreen is important. Sunglasses are also useful, especially if you are going to be running in urban areas where visibility is essential for safety. Sunstroke and dehydration tend to go hand in hand, so as long as you are re-hydrating regularly, you should be able to avoid a case of sunstroke.

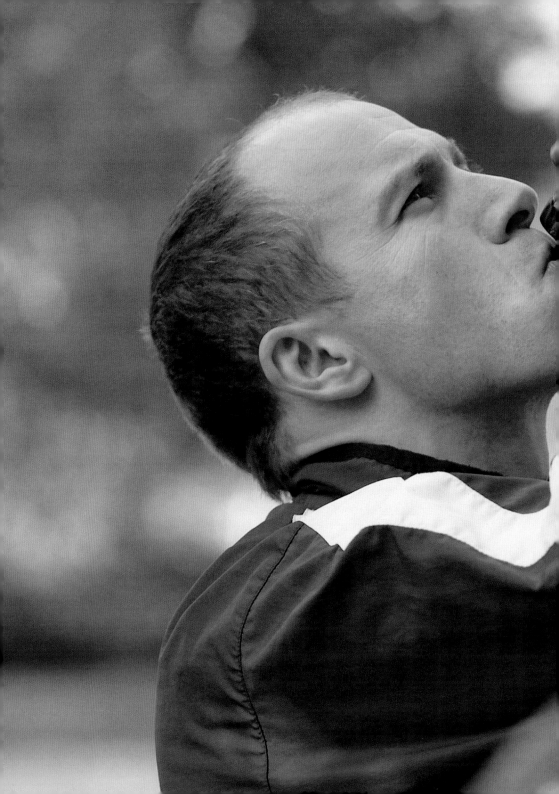

3 Eating & hydration

Running is a demanding activity, requiring good reserves of
energy. Food is the fuel that allows your body to produce
energy. You may want to consider whether making some simple
changes in your diet could help improve your performance.
Alternatively, your priority may be to lose weight and you may
need to adjust your calorie intake. The key is to arm yourself
with some basic knowledge about nutrition; this enables you to
make informed choices about food and build a healthy, varied
and balanced diet that works with your running programme. It
is vital that you keep your body properly hydrated when you're
running. Even slight dehydration can impair your performace,
always replace lost fluid and your body will thank you for it.

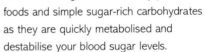
Feeding the machine

As with any endurance activity, performance depends on the right fuel intake. Getting an appropriate nutritional balance can mean the difference between burning out on that long run and blazing through the finish line. With so many differing theories about diet these days, it can be difficult to know what to do. The key is to keep it simple. A healthy diet incorporates protein, carbohydrate and fats in moderate amounts – you need all of these to achieve your fitness goals.

Finding the right mix

Food is your fuel, which will enable you to run. One aspect many people overlook when planning their meals is that eating for fitness is quite different from eating for fat loss. If your training programme is specifically designed to maximise fat loss, your nutritional regime needs to complement it accordingly.

You should base your meals around slow-burning foods (see Glycemic Index, page 42) that are fibre rich and low in sugar. Avoid heavily processed

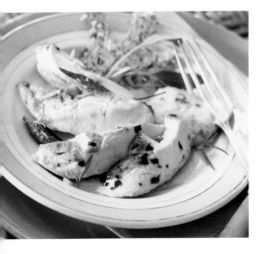

foods and simple sugar-rich carbohydrates as they are quickly metabolised and destabilise your blood sugar levels.

There has been much made by diet industry in recent years of when to eat and though there are a number of conflicting theories, one point holds true: if you take in fewer calories than you put out, you will lose weight. That said, there are certain timing guidelines you can follow to maximise fat loss benefits.

Before a morning run don't eat heavily. A light carbohydrate-based snack, such as a piece of fruit washed down with a glass of water, will aid effort without putting too much strain on your digestive system. If you are running at midday, make sure you have had a substantial breakfast and a small carbohydrate snack 1–2 hours before your workout. If you are exercising in the late afternoon or evening, then a good-sized lunch and a mid-afternoon carbohydrate-filled snack should suffice.

A bit about calories

Most of us would like to shed a few pounds and running can be a great way to burn off calories. However, contrary to popular belief, exercise is just one small part of the weight-loss process. Monitoring food intake is more important. Calorie counting is not necessary, but being aware of the calorie content in the foods you eat is imperative. Your calorie burn will vary daily, so you need to adjust your food intake to account for your activity level. Looking closely at your nutrition and making the necessary changes is the key to attaining your fitness goals.

Remember: food is fuel. When you eat, your body uses the calories from what you have consumed to provide it with energy. In order to lose weight, you need to create a calorie deficit, i.e. eat less than you burn. Men generally need to consume more calories than women, due to the amount of muscle mass a man carries. The more muscle you have, the more calories you will require to preserve that muscle.

Calories and running

Research suggests that the higher the intensity of an activity, the greater the energy coming from carbohydrate rather than fat. This is why running for fat loss involves more long, moderate intensity sessions, while running for cardiovascular conditioning involves high intensity intervals and shorter sessions. Ideally, a balanced training programme will combine both strategies, but for heavy, out-of-condition exercisers, it is best to focus on normalising body weight before going into intense interval work.

Metabolic Rate

Each of us is physically different. Our bodies are unique in many ways – from the rate at which we process nutrients to the amount of energy we use while running. One way our bodies differ individually is in metabolic rate. Resting Metabolic Rate (RMR) is basically the number of calories you burn just by living 24 hours a day, 7 days a week. The higher your RMR, the more calories you will burn at rest.

Everyone has a friend who can eat anything without it having any effect. Likewise, we all know someone who can just look at a bag of chips and put on weight. It all comes down to RMR; whatever your RMR is, that determines how quickly you will gain or lose weight. If you have a slow RMR it doesn't mean you can't lose weight, it just means that you have to work harder than someone with a higher RMR. Though RMR is genetic, there are things you can do to increase it.

Your RMR makes up between 60–80 per cent of your Metabolic Rate (MR). The other 20–40 per cent comes from the work you do, your lifestyle and your activity level. The more physically demanding your job and the more often you work out or participate in sport, the more calories you will burn on a daily basis. On the other hand, consume more calories than your MR, and you will gradually put on weight.

Here are three ways to boost your RMR and MR:

▶ Increase the amount of lean tissue (muscle mass). The bigger your engine, the more calories you burn when your engine is idling. An extra pound of muscle burns an additional 50 calories per day, that's 18,000 extra calories per year.
▶ Be more active. Your metabolism is raised by exercise or general activity. You will burn significantly more calories if you maintain an active lifestyle than if you spend your days sitting in front of the TV or a behind a desk
▶ Eat small meals often. The digestion of food accounts for between 7–13 per cent of your metabolism, as eating speeds up the metabolism due to the energy needed to digest a meal.

Working out your RMR

To get an estimate of your own resting metabolic rate put your details through this equation.

Women 661 + (4.38 x weight/lb) +   **Men** 661 + (6.24 x weight/lb) +
(4.38 x height/in) – (4.7 x age) = RMR   (12.7 x height/in) – (6.9 x age) = RMR

Activity Multiplier Now that you have an estimate of your resting metabolic rate, you can determine how many calories you need each day to meet your bodyweight goals. To calculate your daily caloric requirement, you need to add on the number of calories you burn through exercise or the work that you do. For example, an office worker will burn fewer calories a day than a postman.

Multiply your RMR by one of the following:
Sedentary activity/work   x 1.15   (completely still).
Light activity/work   x 1.3   (normal everyday activity).
Moderately active/work   x 1.4   (exercise 3 times a week).
Very active/work   x 1.6   (exercise 4 times a week).
Extremely active/work   x 1.8   (exercise 6–7 times a week).

Sample Metabolic Profile Female, 140 lb, 35, 5 ft 5 in
By plugging in the correct variables to the above RMR calculation we find:

661+ (4.38 x 140 lbs) + (4.38 x 65 inches) – (4.7 x 35 years) = RMR
661 + 613.2 + 284.7 – 164.5 = 1394 calories

To calculate her overall caloric consumption, we plug RMR into the activity equations:
Sedentary: 1394.4 x 1.15 = 1603.56 calories burned.
Light activity/work: 1394.4 x 1.3 = 1812.72 calories burned.
Moderate activity/work: 1394.4 x 1.4 = 1952.16 calories burned.

Nutrition: the basics

To build a balanced nutritional platform, you're going to need the basics. It is difficult to separate the misinformation from the truth these days. One moment we are hearing that carbohydratess are the main offenders, the next week it is fats. One friend will tell you that a high-protein diet worked wonders for their figure, while another will swear by vegetarianism. The easiest way to wade through the 'expert' advice is to simply learn the basic science of nutrition. Once you have the facts, you can make an informed personal decision about how best to eat for your goals.

Carbohydrates

Carbohydrates have been getting a complete hammering by the press over the past few years. Misunderstandings about their effects, weight-loss fads like high protein diets, and general ignorance about body chemistry, have resulted in a lot of popular confusion. However, carbohydrates are the key nutritional source for athletes.

Carbohydrates exist in many different forms so it is a matter of picking the healthy varieties best suited to your training needs. Generally speaking, they fall into four different categories: fruit, vegetables, alcohol and starches (potatoes, pasta, rice and bread). When it comes to the starches and the spirits, obviously moderation is key, but trying to train without a balance of healthy fruit, vegetables and wholegrains is simply not sustainable. Even those fast-burning carbs, like white rice and cereal bars, have their place. Because they are converted into energy quickly, they're great for an energy boost during or immediately after training. Their fast-burning chemistry means that you can refuel a lot more quickly, turning a tired workout into a sweat-filled success. Carbohydrate provides the main source of energy for the muscles. Unlike other nutrients, carbs can be used in the absence of oxygen, making them the body's first resource when immediate fuel is required. Carbohydrate is stored in three locations in the body: the liver, the muscle

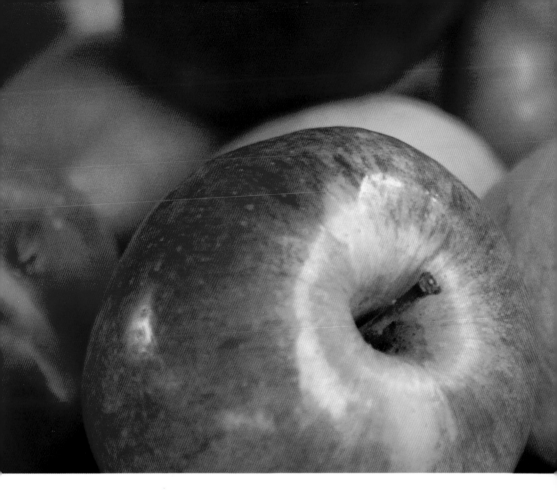

and the blood. In the blood it circulates as glucose, while in the liver and muscle it is stored as glycogen. Glycogen has to be stored with water. Each gram of glycogen requires about 3 g (0.1 oz) water for adequate storage, making it very bulky as an energy store. Unlike fat, which the body can hoard in limitless amounts, the body (e.g. a 70 kg/154 lb man) can only hold around 450 g (1 lb) of glycogen (about 2,000 calories).

The Glycemic Index (GI)

Recent public interest in the Glycemic Index has made carbohydrate the topic of much discussion. The Glycemic Index ranks carbohydrate foods on the basis of how quickly they raise the body's blood sugar levels. Carbohydrates that enter the bloodstream most quickly have the highest Glycemic Index with a ranking of 100, and those entering the bloodstream more slowly have a lower Glycemic Index. Foods that have a low Glycemic Index are absorbed

GIs		
High GI foods	**Moderate GI foods**	**Low GI foods**
White bread	Basmati rice	Apples
White rice	Carrots	Kidney beans
Brown Rice	Spaghetti	Chick peas
Soft drinks	Banana	Pears
Sweet corn	Baked Beans	Yogurt
Potato	Muesli	Plums
Honey	Peas	
Cornflakes		

more slowly, giving a more sustained release of energy, which, in turn, stabilises blood sugar. According to recent research from the University of Sydney in Australia, foods that have a low Glycemic Index will keep you exercising for up to 20 minutes longer than faster burning, high GI foods.

Fat

Not all fat is bad fat. In fact, fat is a highly valuable substance with many different and important roles within the body. Aside from being the most concentrated form of energy, providing the body with more than twice the energy of carbohydrate or protein, certain types of fat can help to protect us against disease. According to researche, by eating a handful of nuts every day, women could nearly halve their risk of coronary disease. Therefore, eating the right fats is just as important as eliminating the bad fats.

Fats can be separated into three groups: essential (polyunsaturates), non-essential (saturated), and monounsaturated fats. Non-essential or saturated fat is what we tend to think of as 'bad' fat. Once ingested, this kind of fat will either be stored by the body or used for energy. Essential or polyunsaturated fats, on the other hand, help to keep us healthy. They are used by the brain and nerves to optimise function; they assist in balancing our hormone levels; they boost immunity and even promote healthy skin. Good sources of essential fats come from seeds such as flax or pumpkin seeds and fish such as mackerel, salmon and tuna. Monounsaturated fat fits between saturated fats and polyunsaturated fats and includes olive oil, avocados and nuts. While the foods high in this type of fat are not as good for the body as those full of essential fat, they are nowhere near as bad for you as items high in saturated fat.

Protein

Research has shown that protein fills you up faster than any other food type. Foods high in protein also require more energy to be expended during digestion, so you end up burning more calories as you process the food.

Protein is an important nutrient because it makes up part of every cell structure in the human body. Protein is necessary for growth of new tissue and repair of damaged tissue. A ready supply of protein is needed on a daily basis to maintain tissue and make thousands of different enzymes within the body. Protein is used as an energy back-up system if glycogen levels become in short supply. Protein is not stored in the same way as carbohydrate and fat it is stored in the form of muscle and organ tissue.

Proteins are made up of smaller units called amino acids. There are 20 amino acids of which 12 are non-essential (those which the body is capable of making). The other eight essential amino acids cannot be produced by the body and can only be supplied through healthy eating. Some foods contain

Benefits of Healthy Fats

- ▶ Energy reserve (1 g/0.3 oz of fat = 9 calories of energy)
- ▶ Protection of vital organs
- ▶ Insulation
- ▶ Transports the fat soluble vitamins A, D, E and K
- ▶ Structure of cell membranes

all eight essential amino acids. These are mostly derived from animals: meat, fish, eggs, milk and dairy products. Other foods such as cereals, nuts, pulses and seeds also contain protein, but not a full complement of amino acids.

Energy values of key nutrients

Carbohydrate (1 g/0.3 oz) = 4.5 calories.
Protein (1 g/0.3 oz) = 4.5 calories.
Fat (1 g/0.3 oz) = 9 calories.
Alcohol (1 g/0.3 oz) = 7 calories.

Getting the balance right

Your energy intake needs to comprise of a combination of fats, carbohydrates and proteins.

▶ Fat: 15–25 per cent
▶ Carbs: 55–65 per cent
▶ Protein: 15–25 per cent

Based on your metabolic rate calculations it is possible to apply this framework to designing a daily nutritional plan that will supply you with the energy and nutrients to meet your running goals.

Vitamins and minerals

Vitamins and minerals do not provide energy; they are needed in certain quantities for good health and general wellbeing.

It is important to note that vitamins and minerals interact, working together to perform a role within the body and very rarely operating in isolation. An individual's requirement will differ according to their age, sex, activity level and body chemistry. A balanced diet, rich in unprocessed and fresh foods is likely to give you the necessary vitamins and minerals.

Vitamins

These are required in tiny amounts for growth, health and physical wellbeing. They have a role in energy production and exercise performance as well as involvement in the functioning of the immune, hormonal and nervous systems. Our bodies are unable to make vitamins so these must be provided by the food we eat.

Minerals

Minerals cannot be made in the body so they must be obtained through diet. They have a multitude of functions within the body including controlling fluid balance in the tissues, muscle contractions, nerve function, enzyme secretions, healthy bones and teeth and the formation of red blood cells.

The importance of variety

When you run, you place stress on the body and it responds by producing free radicals, toxic molecules that damage healthy cells by destablising their normal structures. Unless dealt with, free radicals slowly destroy the body. Antioxidants are the molecules that combat free radical damage. A select group of vitamins, antioxidants like beta-carotene and Vitamin A are found in healthy foods, like fruit and veg, and can help your body to repair toxic breakdown. Therefore, maintaining correct nutrition during training is essential. Getting the right balance of foods will ensure you have enough antioxidants to destroy the free radicals.

Free radicals and antioxidants

Free radicals are formed by exposure to things like pollution, tobacco smoke, alcohol, insecticides, radiation, and chemicals. They can even be caused by exposure to excessive amounts of sunlight. Additionally, eating a high-fat diet or regularly engaging in strenuous exercise can cause the excessive and uncontrolled production of free radicals.

Free radicals can have devastating health effects. A high concentration of free radicals can cause the 'bad' (LDL) cholesterol to stick to the walls of your arteries, increasing your risk of a stroke or heart attack. Free radicals also react with important cellular components such as DNA or the cell membrane, leading to cell malfunction and death. Normally, our bodies are designed to handle free radicals by combating them with antioxidants derived from healthy foods, but if antioxidants are unavailable, or if the free-radical production becomes excessive, damage can occur. It is particularly important to note that free radical damage accumulates with age. But before you panic and decide to adopt radical lifestyle changes, it is good to know that there are simple, subtle ways we can reduce free radical production in our bodies. By controlling destructive behaviours like the poor diet choices and excessive high intensity exercise that lead to increased free radical production, we can significantly reduce their levels within our bodies. Moderate exercise and an antioxidant-rich diet are ideal ways we can help our bodies 'deactivate' free radicals before they cause harm.

Examples of antioxidants

The principal antioxidants are vitamin E, vitamin C and beta-carotene (a precursor to vitamin A). Vitamin A and beta-carotene are most abundantly found in colourful fruits and vegetables such as carrots, apricots, dark green leafy vegetables, red peppers, sweet potatoes, and blue-green algae. Vitamin E is found in nuts, wholegrains, vegetable oils and, to a lesser extent, in fruits and vegetables. Vitamin C is found in most fruits and vegetables, especially blackcurrants, berries, broccoli, cabbage, citrus fruits, peppers, kale, kiwi fruits, papaya, spinach, tomatoes, and watercress.

Hydration and running

We don't drink enough water. It is no laughing matter: dehydration impairs physiological function, hampers performance and increases the risk of heat exhaustion. According to a recent study, one-third of British adults don't drink enough water. Rather, they tend to opt for caffeine-based drinks, that are actually counterproductive to hydration, having a diuretic effect on the body.

Losing hydration

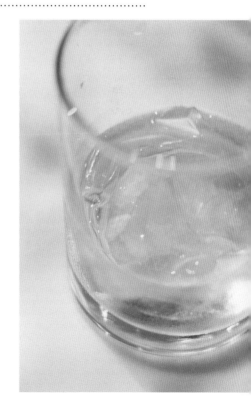

You may not notice how much fluid/water you're losing, especially when you're running outdoors, because it evaporates off the skin in the breeze. Don't underestimate the amount of fluid you will need to replace, particularly in hot weather. Rates of water loss can be up to 1 litre (1¾ pints) per hour, so keep water on hand. Water hydration backpacks are extremely useful (see page 31), since no real effort is required to drink from them. The equivalent of a 2 per cent decrease in body weight increases the stress on the body resulting in impaired performance. Preventing dehydration will allow you to work longer and harder.

How dehydrated you become depends on the intensity of your run, the duration and the weather conditions. Running hard for 1–2 hours in hot weather conditions is going to put you most at risk.

When beginning any exercise programme, it is essential to increase your hydration levels to compensate for fluid loss during exercise. Make a habit of having a glass of water prior to running.

Things to remember about dehydration
▶ Slight dehydration can and will affect performance.
▶ Headaches might be caused by dehydration.

Energy drinks

Losing fluid during a run is one thing, but losing sodium (salt) is a different ball game altogether. Water is not the only thing depleted by training, especially during longer sessions. As you exercise, your body tries to maintain a constant core temperature by increasing the rate at which you sweat – however, the downside is you lose sodium as well as fluid. The longer you go on, the more salt you lose.

Electrolyte (salt and mineral) and energy (carbohydrate) replacement is essential and can come in the form of sports drinks. Sometimes it can be difficult to eat solid fuels while running. Ideally you will wear a customised water carrier belt with two water bottle holders – one filled with water and the other with a sports drink. If you are only consuming water you run the risk of diluting the sodium concentration in your blood.

You don't have to spend heaps of cash on the latest sports drink. A simple orange squash can do the trick and at only a fraction of the cost. Just remember to dilute it: 1 part squash to 3 parts water. For a variation add a little salt (1-1.5 g/0.3 oz) to make it an electrolyte drink.

Seasonal considerations

In hot weather, you can sweat up to 2 litres (3½ pints) of water per hour. Make sure that you carry water/energy drink with you during summer runs.

Women and running nutrition

Calcium

One of the most important minerals in a woman's diet, calcium is essential for maintaining healthy bones and may even prevent high blood pressure and colon cancer. Eating habits have a big impact on bone mineral density. Make sure that you ingest 1,000–1,500 mg per day of calcium as well as Vitamins D, A, C, B6 and K.

Bone density

Any exercise activity will strengthen bones to some degree. However, in order to achieve the best results, a balanced diet is essential. A good dose of calcium can be found in dairy products, leafy greens, nuts and seafood. And be careful, as excessive alcohol and protein intake can block calcium absorption.

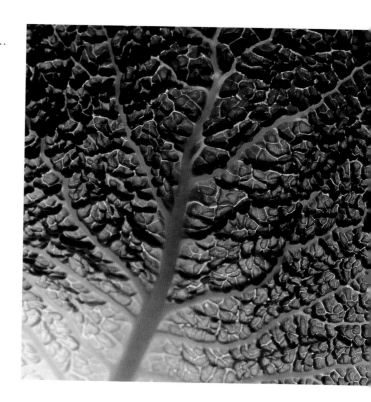

Monitoring your nutrition: tools and tips

Depending on your goals, you may need to invest more or less time in this area. If weight is not an issue, then being careful to maintain a healthy, clean and balanced diet is probably all you need to do. Make sure you fuel up properly before long runs, carry adequate liquids and eat a balance of protein, fats and carbs in every meal. If, however, you are struggling with weight loss, maintenance or gain, or finding your energy levels lagging, take a closer look at your nutrition. There are several ways of doing this:

Calculate your metabolism

Using the formula given earlier in this chapter (see page 39), figure out your Resting Metabolic Rate (RMR). Factor in your activity level and any additional exercise you may be doing.

If you are finding yourself tired or even depressed, it may be that you are taking in fewer healthy calories than you need to sustain your level of activity. If the majority of your daily intake is coming from highly processed foods, sugars, or other 'empty' sources, though you might be meeting the daily requirement numerically, your body is still not getting the nutrients it needs to restore its systems and recover adequately. Over time you will be left feeling tired, cranky and weak. In fact, it is possible in this era of fast food and processing, to be at a normal weight, or even quite overweight and malnourished, contradictory as it may sound.

If weight loss is your goal, assessing your metabolic rate and then designing a balanced meal plan to meet your weight loss goals is the key to success. Considering that 450g (1 lb) of fat is worth approximately 3,500 calories, to lose approximately 1 kg (2 lbs) a week (the safest rate for ensuring long-term success) you will need to aim for a weekly deficit of

3,500 to 7,000 calories. It is very important that your daily caloric intake does not fall below your RMR, as this will actually cause your RMR to slow down, not to mention leave you hungry, weak and prone to success-sabotaging binges. It may be advisable to meet with a nutritionist before starting any modified diet, as they can advise you on the best strategies for healthy weight loss and assist you in developing a balanced eating plan.

Keep a log

In the same way that a training log can help you spot weaknesses in your exercise programme, a food diary can highlight the nutritional deficiencies or indulgences that are sabotaging your success. By tracking your intake, you can easily spot the negative patterns (like overindulging in the afternoons or eating late at night) that are slowing your progress. You might find that not having adequate protein at lunch is the constant factor preceding a lacklustre evening workout or that skipping breakfast is the common element on days when you overeat in the evenings. Keeping track of dietary patterns is a useful way to retrain oneself nutritionally, leading to a better quality of life down the line.

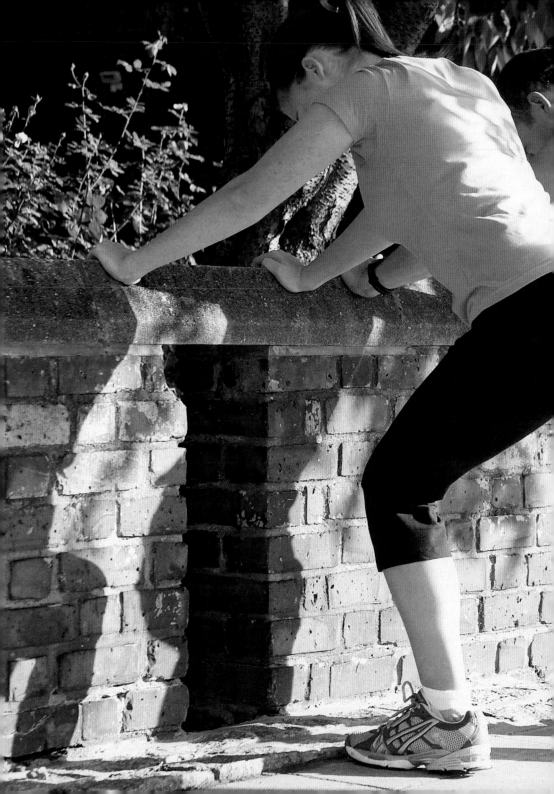

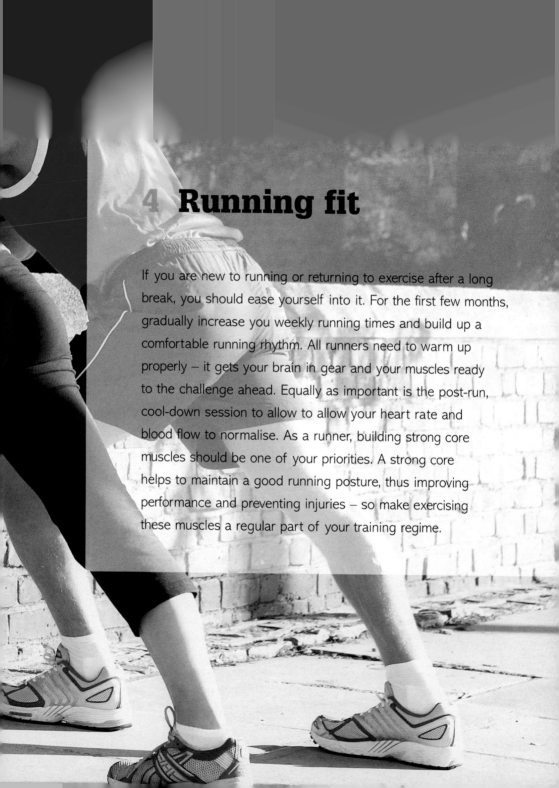

4 Running fit

If you are new to running or returning to exercise after a long
break, you should ease yourself into it. For the first few months,
gradually increase you weekly running times and build up a
comfortable running rhythm. All runners need to warm up
properly – it gets your brain in gear and your muscles ready
to the challenge ahead. Equally as important is the post-run,
cool-down session to allow to allow your heart rate and
blood flow to normalise. As a runner, building strong core
muscles should be one of your priorities. A strong core
helps to maintain a good running posture, thus improving
performance and preventing injuries – so make exercising
these muscles a regular part of your training regime.

Start right

You've made the decision to start a running programme, but feel slightly uneasy about how to begin. There is one universal rule that applies to anyone just starting out or those returning to exercise after a long break: gently ease yourself into the activity. If you haven't run for many years or if this is your first time, it might be safer to start walking before you even attempt to run. You can gradually move into jogging and running as your body acclimatises. A walk/run programme is an effective way to build fitness, and there is no reason to push yourself to meet unrealistic expectations that can potentially cause injury.

In Chapter 6, I will take you through the guidelines for designing your personal running regimen, but before we get into specifics and personal goals there are a few general points to bear in mind. Basically, when structuring a run, one tends to aim for either time or distance. The framework you choose is up to the individual. For beginners, it is a lot easier to build your run around time, because it's very hard to gauge distances when you're running in parks or along streets. If you go for distance, you tend to worry about speed in order to complete the distance as quickly as possible. So at the start, perhaps focus on building time.

As a beginner, running out of steam quickly is pretty much inevitable. In fact, it is common for beginners to feel disheartened when they start out. The shortness of breath, wheezing and gasping can be enough to put someone off running for life. But there are ways to soften the impact, to make the transition to a higher level of fitness a smooth one.

The first few runs are always the hardest – believe me, it does get easier and more enjoyable as your fitness level increases. Once you start to run and notice how much better you feel, you'll never look back.

Keep listening to your body. If you're gasping for air and feeling dizzy or light-headed, then take the pace down a notch or walk until you have recovered. You will find that the more you respect your natural fitness limits, the more quickly your body will adapt and allow you to reach your goals.

There are many factors that determine how you should start your running career.

- ▶ Your age.
- ▶ Your weight.
- ▶ Your previous health condition.
- ▶ Your current lifestyle.

If you are unsure if you are physically fit enough to start a training programme it is advisable to visit your doctor to assess your readiness.

How to ease into it – the run/walk programme

The first 3 months should be dedicated to adding gradually to the amount of time spent running. A long run at the weekend and 2–3 runs during the week is a good way to start. Once you can complete a run comfortably for around 30+ minutes, it's time to start introducing some speed work and variety into your training schedule. Within 3 months, there is no reason why you should not be running for sustained periods of 1+ hours. So in the beginning, don't worry at all about distance, simply go out and gradually build up your time.

Running technique

If you have ever watched a running event you will have witnessed some of the weird and wonderful styles of running out there. Some styles look downright awkward and uncomfortable, but they are still effective. Technique is very subjective and sometimes you will find that the athletes with the weirdest running styles carry the fewest injuries.

However, on the flipside, bad running styles can lead to a whole plethora of injuries. Daily living can also affect your running form over time: sitting down for hours on end shortens the hip flexors and deactivates core muscles; sitting cross-legged rotates the hips; and working at a computer promotes a forward head posture an/or rounded shoulders. Good posture is essential for an efficient running stride.

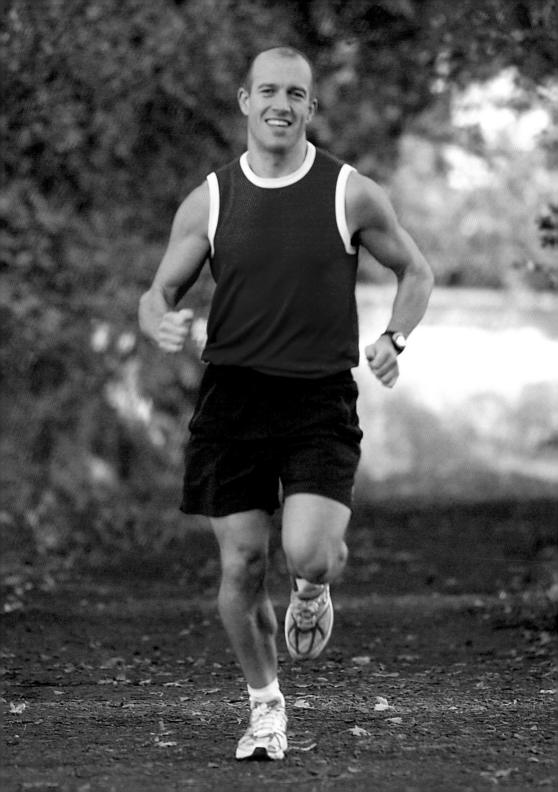

Key Pointers on Technique and Posture

▶ Maintain some abdominal and gluteal (bottom) tension.
▶ Relax shoulders to eliminate tension.
▶ Relax hands, don't clench them.
▶ Look forward, not down at your feet.
▶ Move the arms rhythmically across the body.
▶ Relax your facial muscles.
▶ Adopt an upright posture.

Lastly, as you move, notice how your feet are meeting the ground. Landing hard on your heels can cause a variety of problems and force your legs to absorb too much forward momentum. Land softly on your heels and roll forward on to your toes.

Pace

Running is about rhythm. The cadence of your step should be fluid and comfortable. Strides should be consistent and uniform, which can be difficult when running outdoors. If you are alternating between different speed intervals, you should find your pace within each level. Maintaining proper posture will assist you in keeping your pace steady.

A good technique for assessing the suitability of your pace is the 'talk test'. If you can't hold a conversation during the first half of your run, then you are probably going too fast. If you are doing an 'easy' run then you should be able to maintain a conversation throughout. If it's a 'hard fast' run and you can talk, then you're not pushing yourself enough.

Running outside vs. running inside

One of the strongest selling points running has is its simplicity. You don't need a fancy gym membership, a ton of gear or complicated equipment to perform effectively. That said, consistency is essential if your fitness is to improve, and so choosing an environment that appeals to you is important.

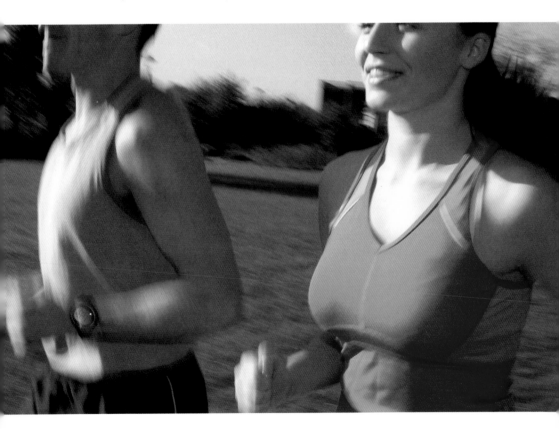

If you prefer the gym, there is no reason to force yourself to head outside. However, your body will benefit from exercising over different terrain and running outside is a great way to relieve stress and lighten your mood. Relying entirely on the treadmill at your local gym can also lead to failure, as when one isn't available you'll be inclined to forego your run. For all these reasons, my advice is that you force yourself to train outside at least once or twice a week.

Running outdoors accelerates conditioning of the ligaments in your lower body, making you more responsive and improving your agility. Outdoor workouts help to develop balance and work the muscles and ligaments around your ankle joints. Running on uneven ground strengthens the joints in a variety of ways, unlike a treadmill workout.

Outdoor running is a more free and natural form of exercise. If you are concerned about the long-term impact of running on a hard road surface, running in woodland or grassy areas is kinder on the joints and a great way to avoid the traffic. If you can find a good route, somewhere scenic, then you will never want to run indoors again

On the other hand, treadmills are a good place to start because you can control the pace and you don't have to battle the elements.

Quick comparison – indoor running vs. outdoor running

Indoor

Weather protected

Fewer safety concerns

Convenient and affordable

Limited gear required – just shoes

Easier to achieve a

consistent pace

Outdoor

Fresh air enhances the

feeling of wellbeing

Ever-changing environment

to keep it fun

Variety of terrain for enhanced

training benefits

Looking after your running body

It is widely accepted that prevention is far better than cure. With this in mind, let's turn to the various preventative techniques proven to decrease the potential for injury.

Warming up

In Chapter 2, I reviewed the basics of warming up and easing into your running programme. The thing to remember is that the body needs to be introduced into a workout gradually. The first 5 minutes of any run should consist of walking to increase blood flow to the large muscle groups. As the blood flow increases, the muscles will be able to access more oxygen and nutrients to perform well. A common mistake for first timers is to set off far too quickly – and within a very short space of time be completely shattered. Your body needs time to get enough oxygen to the working muscles. Instead, warm up gradually by walking at an increasing pace for up to 5 minutes.

Warming up achieves four things: it moves blood to where it is needed; it lifts core temperature; it gets your brain in gear and ready for your run; and it allows muscles enough time to get warm and gradually push through to their full range of motion.

Once you get going, an easy way to tell if your mind is driving you to ignore your body's signals is to notice how your feet are hitting the pavement. If you are stamping, driving your feet into the pavement, then it's time for a break. And remember, if you think that the pace is too quick, then

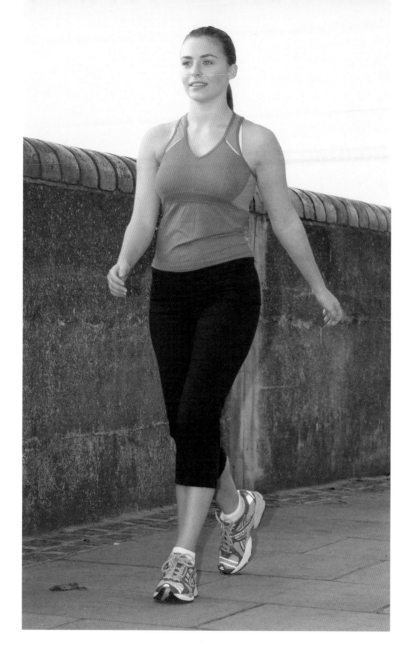

it probably is, so slow down. It's not a race after all. Be assured, you will get quicker over a relatively short period of time.

Having walk breaks is totally acceptable and sensible. Use them as much as you need and don't wait until you're totally out of breath to use them. Follow the run/walk programme on page 123.

Cooling down

There are many reasons for a cool-down session after a workout. The cooling down process allows the body to make the gradual transition from a high heart rate to a near resting heart rate. Cooling down also allows blood flow to normalise around the body.

When running, your heart pumps oxygenated blood to your legs, where it's needed most, and stopping suddenly can cause the blood to pool in the legs, slowing circulation and the removal of lactic acid and carbon dioxide. The cooling down process allows your blood flow to normalise. It is also a good time to stretch, as warm muscles are more pliable than cold ones.

Stretching

Stretching tends to be the most neglected part of the exercise routine. For those of us pressed to fit our workout into a busy schedule, it can seem a waste of time and energy – a luxury one adds on when time permits. But getting into the habit of a stretch routine is a must. Remember, flexibility is one of the many components of fitness, along with strength, cardiovascular, agility, stamina and endurance. If time is short, then make sure that you at least go through a basic sequence of the main stretches. If your schedule is more flexible, then spend between 10 and 15 minutes stretching in front of the TV.

Consistent stretching will keep muscles looser, meaning injuries should be less frequent. It will also help you to run faster. The bottom line is, most of us need to stretch more.

To make the process more comfortable and effective:

▶ Make sure that your muscles are sufficiently warm before you stretch them.
▶ Have a hot bath or sit in front of a fire – a great way to heat the body before you stretch.

Stretching and the workout

On the whole, stretching should be comfortable and pain free. Unfortunately you will find that this isn't always the case. Stretching through tight muscles can be a real challenge. When you can, maintain a constant tension on the muscle, hold for 30+ seconds and avoid any rapid bouncing or jerky movements. Use very small increments backwards and forwards to increase or decrease the stretch.

Pre-exercise Stretching is not always necessary before going out for a run. Always make sure that you gradually warm your body up. If you need to stretch a particular muscle, then stop and stretch out. Though the pre-run stretch is optional, the post-run stretch is not.

Post-exercise After a run, it's just as important to stretch out the upper body as the legs. The chest, shoulders and arms work hard, too. If you experience tightness in your upper body while running, one way of relaxing the arms is just to let them hang down by your sides and shake them out.

How to stretch properly Take long, slow breaths when you stretch. When first stretching a muscle, it might seem particularly tight. However, after about 15–20 seconds, the muscle will desensitise and you should be able to increase the stretch a little further. Always exhale as you increase the stretch, exhaling helps you to move into it. Focus on the muscles that seem to be the tightest and, if necessary, go back to them, stretching them a second or third time in order to equal out the flexibility.

How long should I hold a stretch? The general consensus is that holding stretches for longer periods will produce greater ranges of motion. In fact, current research suggests that one should hold stretches for up to 90 seconds. Holding stretches for 2+ minutes will also elicit positive results.

It is important to stretch muscles when they are warm. Stretching after running is performed to elongate those muscles that have spent the last 30+ minutes contracting. Each stretch needs to be held for minimum of 30 seconds. Remember: the stretch should feel uncomfortable but not painful.

The stretches

Lower back Lie down on your back. Place your right hand out to the side. Bring your right knee up and place your left hand on the knee. Breathe out and pull the knee over and across your body. Repeat on the other side.

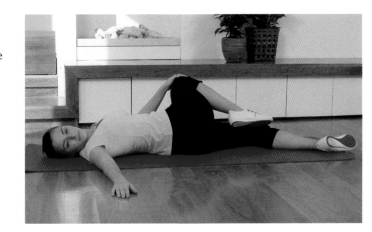

Hamstring Lie down on your back and bend both knees, keeping your feet on the floor. Lift one leg up and link your fingers around the calf muscle. Keeping your head in contact with the floor gently ease the leg towards you. If this is not possible, then use a towel (as shown). Do not let the other knee drift to the side. Keep the knee very slightly bent as you stretch the hamstring. Repeat with the other leg.

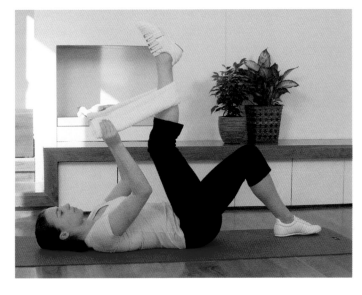

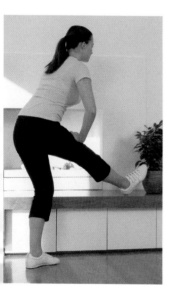 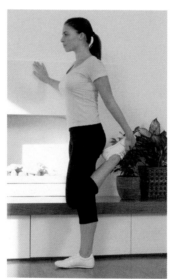 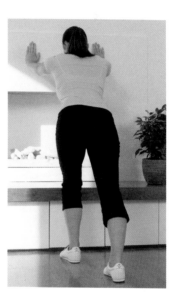

Standing hamstring Standing tall, place one leg on to a raised surface such as a seat or low wall. Keep your standing knee slightly bent and then pivot forward from the hips maintaining a straight back as you do so. Repeat on the other side.

Quadriceps Standing, take one foot up behind your bottom. Hold the heel into your bottom, and then slowly tuck your tail under to reduce the curve in your lower back. This will also increase the stretch in the quadriceps. Hold on to something for balance if you need to. Repeat with the other leg.

Calf Facing a wall, take one foot behind you. Keeping both feet pointing forwards, push the back heel into the ground. Keep the line between your heel and shoulder as straight as possible. Repeat with the other leg.

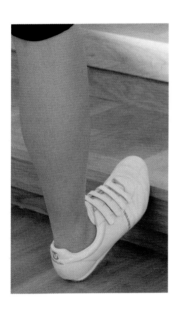 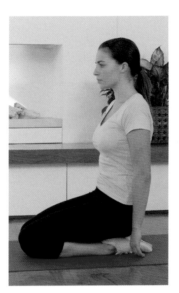 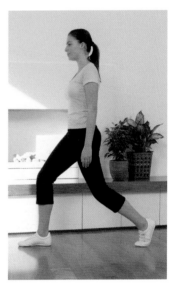

Lower calf Place your foot on the edge of a step/book and bend the knee forward. Repeat with the other leg.

Shins Kneel on the floor. Gently sit back down on to your heels, keeping your back straight.

Hip flexors Place your right foot a good distance out in front of you with your knee bent. Tuck your tail under, so that you feel the abdominals engage. Now lunge gently forward making sure that the right knee does not travel too far over the right foot. Push forward with the left hip while maintaining straight hips. Repeat with the other leg.

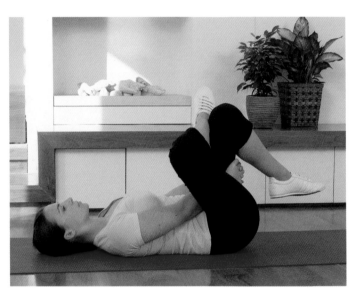

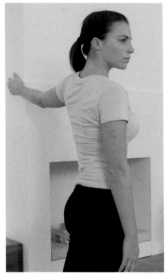

Glutes Lie on your back with your knees bent at 90 degrees and your feet on the floor. Take the right foot and rest the ankle across the left knee. Pull the left knee towards you so you feel the stretch in the right glute. Repeat with the other leg.

Chest Stand and place one hand in the frame of a door. Now turn your body away from the hand and feel the stretch through the chest. Repeat with the other arm.

Cross-training

To ensure you don't overstrain your muscles, combine your routine with other sorts of exercise. Resistance training is particularly important for runners, because building muscle will provide you with added energy and strength for speed and endurance. Swimming, cycling and elliptical training are also good additions to a running programme. When you consistently do the same routine, your body adapts to the required level and no further. By mixing things up with other forms of activity, you will force your system to continue improving, challenging the same muscles to work in different ways. This also lowers the risk of repetitive use injury.

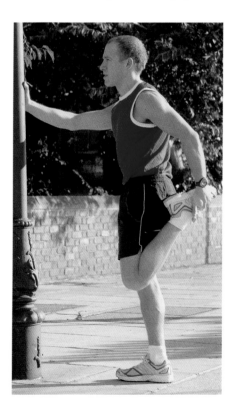

Rest

For beginners, the single greatest cause of injury is pushing yourself beyond your limits. While challenging yourself is an important aspect of building fitness, it can be difficult to know when to push and when to relax. Resting between workouts is absolutely essential if you are to avoid injury. It allows your body to adapt and strengthen in preparation for your next workout. My advice to all runners is to follow a standard run/rest plan when training.

Core strength

There are two basic types of muscle: those that stabilise (holding bones in place) and those that mobilise (move bones). Your deep core muscles are a good example of stabilising muscles. They keep your spine in line, thereby stabilising all the other bones in your skeleton. That is why strong abdominals are the key to good balance and control in motion. Building a strong core will make it easier to maintain good running posture, meaning you will fatigue less quickly over those longer distances.

These days, with our increasingly sedentary lifestyles, the body's core muscles are getting less and less use. With the majority of us spending our days behind desks and our evenings on the couch, it is essential to strengthen these muscle groups through focused training. Adding abdominal and lower back exercises to your daily routine will help you build strong core muscles, preventing injury and improving performance. When the muscles of the core are weak and in a poor condition, additional stress is placed on the surrounding joint structures and muscles. In fact, a high percentage of lower back injuries, and even upper and lower body injuries, stem from a weakness in the core. The exercises on the following pages target a variety of muscle groups throughout your abdominal and lower back regions and have been designed to make your overall core structure stronger.

What is the Core?

Basically, your core is a network of muscles in your torso that provides you with your very own natural corset. There is so much more to abdominals than the six-pack. The deepest muscles within the abdomen are the ones that stabilise the lower back (lumbar spine). These are the transverse abdominis, the pelvic floor and multifidus.

The core provides the essential link between the upper and lower body. Think of it as the body's powerhouse. Lack of use and/or misuse will have an effect on your overall muscle function. In running, it is particularly important to maintain a strong torso, and not just for posture and balance. As your body's energy centre, the core provides the necessary foundations from which the legs can generate the power to run faster and farther. Neglect these central muscles and you will find running a much greater challenge!

Exercising your core muscles

If you think that doing lots of abdominal crunches will reduce the size of your stomach, then think again. Crunches and standard abdominal exercise work only the rectus abdominis, the large muscle located beneath the fat you are storing around your tummy. The muscles you need to be targeting to build core strength are the more deeply set transverse abdominis and internal obliques. Just as important are the lower back and gluteal (bottom) muscles. Along with the abdominals, they form the core and are essential for spine stabilisation. A good core workout must also incorporate the lower back muscles, the paraspinal and deep lumbar muscles.

When you walk, your body moves in a cross-pattern motion with your opposite arm and foot simultaneously moving forward, causing your torso to rotate with each step. To work your core muscles effectively, you need to incorporate exercises that mimic this natural motion. By combining a series of rotational and cross-pattern style abdominal exercises, this programme will maximise impact and give you a really strong set of core muscles.

Things to Remember Quite frequently, core exercises are done far too quickly. Quality is overlooked for quantity. As you follow the exercises described on the following pages, focus on maintaining the form and intensity of each movement, rather than the number of repetitions completed.

Getting started – positioning for your core workout

To effectively target your core muscles, you need to work from a neutral spine position. For many, neutral spine is a very hard position to find. When we lie flat on our backs, our spine moves in a natural curve away from the floor. Neutral spine is this relaxed position. Your back is neither arched nor flat.

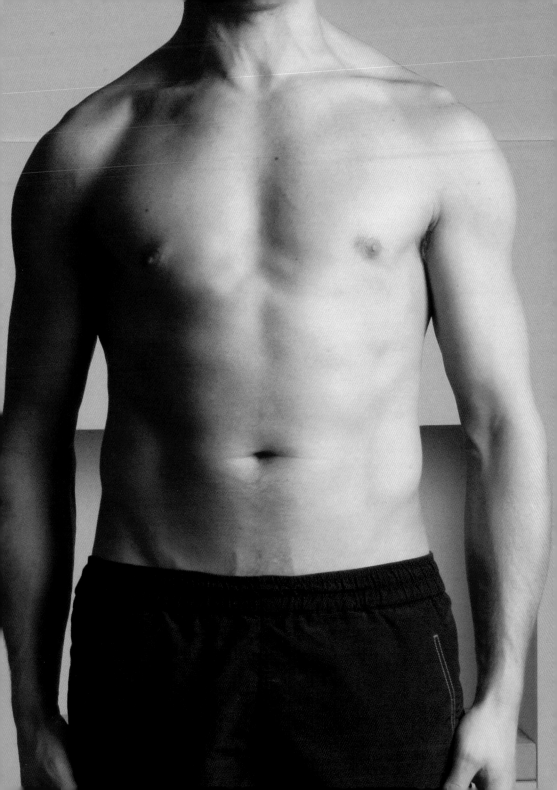

Instead, it is somewhere in between the two. Before beginning any exercise, take a moment to adjust your body and make certain you are working from the correct base.

One of the best ways to find neutral positioning is to lie on your back with your knees bent. Arch your back so you create a tunnel underneath the lower back. Now flatten your back so that there is no tunnel and your spine is pushed firmly into the floor. That's an arched back and a flat back. Now move from flat to arched by using your pelvis. Stop halfway between the two positions so there remains a small natural arch in your lower back. This is neutral spine and in an ideal world all exercises would be performed from this position. In reality, it can be quite a challenge when you are first starting out. Keep with it and eventually you will naturally move into this position for core work.

It's all well and good being able to find your neutral spine position, but the real work is being able to hold it while you perform the exercises. There are several good techniques for holding this neutral spine. Some may work better than others for you. One popular way to keep position is by tightening your pelvic floor. Simply imagine that you are urinating and you need to stop peeing mid-flow, or that you are dying to go to the loo but there is nowhere to go. Next, draw the belly button towards the spine without pushing the lower back into the floor. There, now that should do the trick – or send you running to the loo...

On the following pages there are several tried and tested abdominal exercises. Aim to complete between 10–20 repetitions of each exercise and between 1–2 sets. Beginners should start with 1 set of 10 repetitions, building up as they get stonger.

Floor exercises

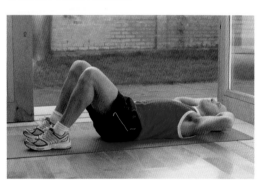

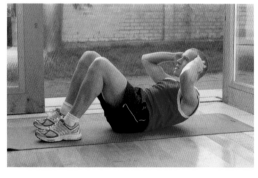

Crunch Lying on your back, activate your pelvic floor and draw your belly button towards your spine without pushing your back into the floor. Place your hands on your temples. Slowly lift your shoulders off the floor contracting the abdominals. Hold at the top position for a count of three and then slowly lower back down to the floor. If your neck hurts, then place a fist between your chin and chest. Try to lift with your shoulders rather than your head.

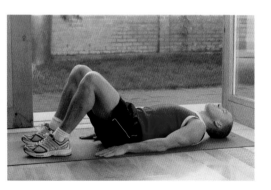

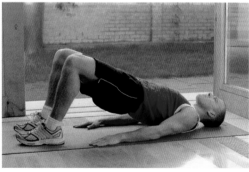

Body Hip Lift and bridge Lie on your back with your arms by your sides and your knees bent. Tighten your abdominals and lift your hips off the floor until your body forms a straight line from your knees to your shoulders. Whilst keeping the glutes and abdominals tight, hold the position for 5–10 seconds before slowly lowering your body back down to the floor.

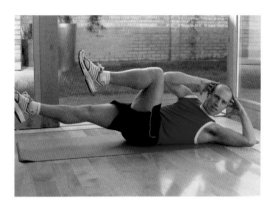

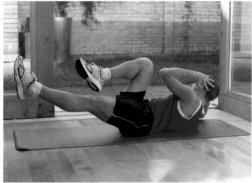

Bicycle crunch Lie on your back with your feet in the air. Alternately move your legs out in front of you as if you were cycling. As you do so, touch the opposite elbow to the opposite knee. Make sure it

is the outside of the elbow that touches the outside of the knee. Pause each time the knee connects with the elbow.

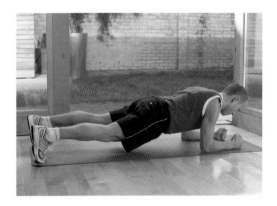

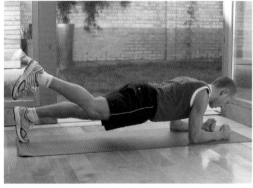

Plank on the mat Kneel on the floor, lie down and position yourself on your elbows. Lift up off your knees so only your toes and forearms are in contact

with the floor. Hold for 30–60 seconds. To make it harder lift one leg off the floor, hold for a pause, then return the foot and then lift the other foot.

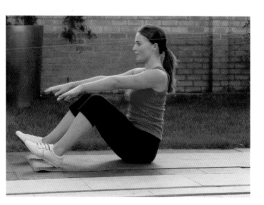 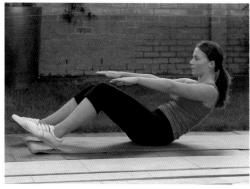

Roll down Start in a seated position with your legs out in front of you and with your knees slightly bent. Place your hands on to your knees and lower your upper body down towards the floor as slowly as you can, one vertebra at a time. Keep the movement as slow as you can.

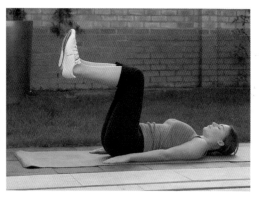 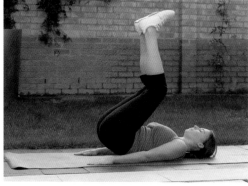

Reverse crunch Lie on your back with your knees up in the air. Then slowly, using your abdominals, pull the knees towards your head without using excessive momentum. Pull in and hold briefly and then slowly lower back to the start position.

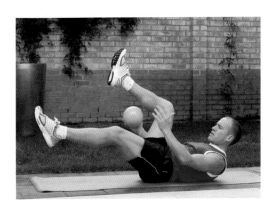 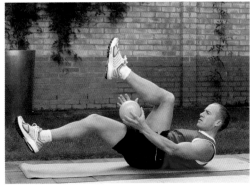

Bicycle Pass the medicine ball in a figure-of-eight pattern in between the legs. To make it slightly harder, lift the head and crunch your abdominals at the same time. Aim to do 50 passes.

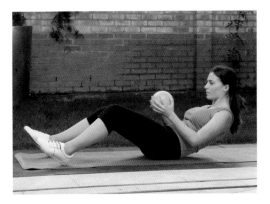 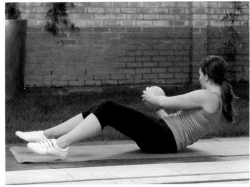

Rolldown twist Sit up with your knees bent. Take hold of the medicine ball, then slowly lower yourself down to the floor to the point where you feel the abdominals engage. Then rotate from side to side with the ball. Aim to do 10–20 rotations.

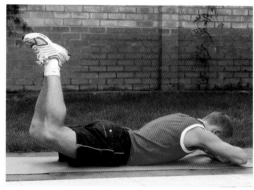

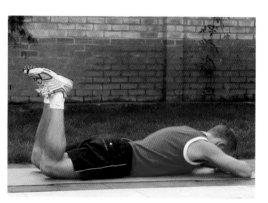

Glutes lift Lie face down on the floor resting your head in your hands. Bend your knees so that the soles of your feet are facing skyward. Tighten your abdominals and lift your knees off the floor, squeezing your buttocks and lower back muscles. You should only be able to lift your knees a couple of inches off the floor. Hold for a second or two, then lower your knees back to the floor.

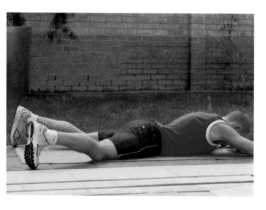

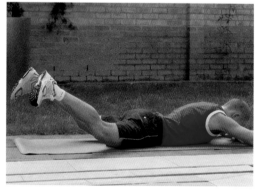

Scissor lift Lie face down on the floor, resting your head in your hands. Spread your legs as wide as you can. Keeping your legs straight, tighten your abdominals and lift both legs off the floor. Hold for a second or two, then lower your legs back to the floor.

Training on a stability ball

Stability ball training has its roots in rehabilitation: it is used by many physical therapists and orthopedic specialists worldwide. Its popularity has grown enormously within the gym and home environments in the last decade due to its versatility and simplicity. Because the ball demands balance, you will work many muscles you never knew you had, offering a fun, safe and highly effective way to exercise. As you quickly find out, you don't just get on the stability ball and begin to exercise. You can try, but you might do more damage than good. Seeking the help of a qualified trainer is always beneficial at the start.

So why use a stability ball? The use of traditional exercise equipment does not necessarily challenge whole groups of muscles in one go and the most important muscles that act as our foundations are often overlooked. The stability ball, on the other hand, adds a new dimension to the exercise: instability. When the body is in an unstable environment, more muscles are recruited to provide the necessary stability and balance. It is the muscles of the core that stabilise the rest of the body and provide the link between the lower and upper body. Having a solid core creates a foundation upon which to perform. When used correctly, stability ball exercise calls upon constant activation of the core.

Using the stability ball and incorporating free-weight exercises is a great way to develop strength in the extremities while training the key core muscles at the same time. Even while training other muscle groups, the abdominal and back musculature is simultaneously working to balance and stabilise the body. Strong postural muscles and proper posture are important for relieving and preventing lower back pain. Training with the ball can improve muscle tone, increase muscular endurance and strength, restore or improve flexibility, enhance spinal stability, complement resistance and aerobic training programmes, help lose weight, and, lastly, improve balance, posture and coordination.

So throw away that ab roller packed neatly underneath the bed. The stability ball is probably the best piece of training equipment you can buy and offers a whole lot more.

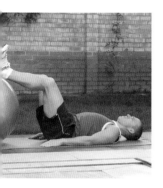 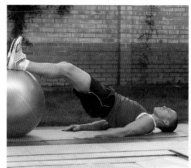 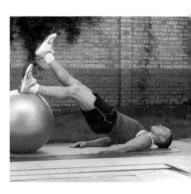

Hip bridge on the ball Lie on your back and place both feet on top of the ball. Push your lower back into the floor and lift your hips off the floor.

Hold for 10 seconds and repeat 10 times. To make the movement harder, lift one leg off the ball when you're in the bridge position.

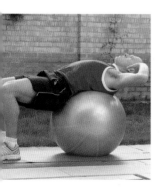 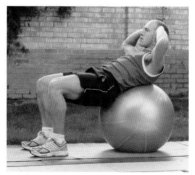 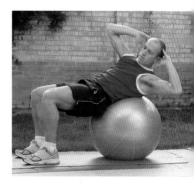

Ball crunch Lie down on top of the ball. Heels should be under your knees and knees should be hip width apart. Place your hips at a lower level than your shoulders to make the movement easier. Keep the base of the spine and the top of your

bottom in contact with the ball at all times. Place fingers next to temples, breath out and curl yourself upwards using your abdominals, keeping the ball motionless. **Ball twist crunch** As above, but add a twisting motion as you curl up.

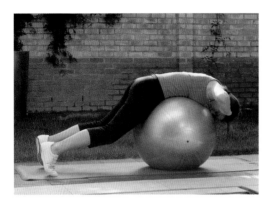

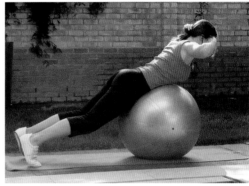

Back extension Roll over the top of the ball keeping your toes in contact with the floor. Place your fingers next to your temples and let your upper body curve around the ball. Tighten your abdominals and slowly lift your upper body off the ball. Keep your eyes looking towards the floor.

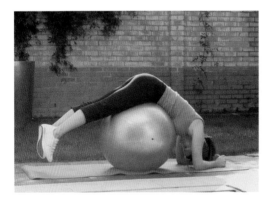

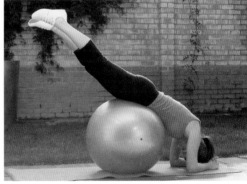

Glute lift Roll right over the ball and rest on to your forearms on the floor. Keeping the legs together tighten your abs and lift both your legs off the floor, squeezing your glutes and lower back.

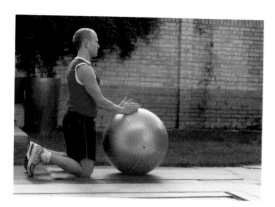

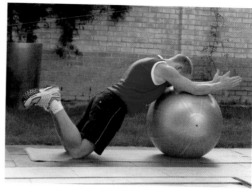

Forward ball roll Kneel behind the ball and place your hands on top of it. Using your knees as a pivot, keeping your core strong, slowly roll the ball forward maintaining a straight line from your shoulder to your knee. Don't go too far. Pull yourself back to the start position.

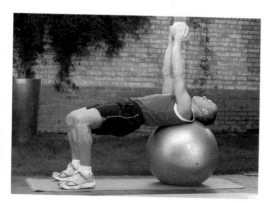

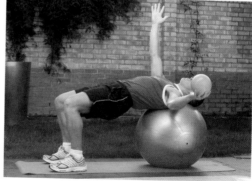

Stability ball rotation Lie on your back on the ball, holding a medicine ball. Walk your feet out until only your shoulders and neck are resting on the ball. Push the medicine ball above your chest. Release into one hand and slowly lower the arm out to the side, keeping the arm as straight as possible, while maintaining tight abdominals.

Weight training – building strength effectively

Running is fine for building endurance and stamina within the leg muscles, but not very good at building long-term strength and power. A well-designed resistance programme will give you a stronger, more powerful lower body and, consequently, greater endurance and stamina for the legs.

Stronger muscles are of definite benefit to runners of all shapes and sizes. The effect of having stronger legs means that you won't become as tired as quickly. You'll be able to run faster, hills will seem easier and it will be possible to sprint at the end of a race.

All runners, be they sprinters or ultra marathoners, will reap benefits from a resistance-based fitness programme.

The benefits of weight training

Using weights will help you achieve a desired body shape, but it also has many other benefits. As your muscles strengthen, physical activity become easier, and because it lowers blood pressure and cholesterol levels, consistent training is also very good for the heart.

Other reasons to lift:
▶ Reduces risk of injury: Your muscles act as shock absorbers to prevent injury from external forces and overuse.
▶ Improved injury rehabilitation: A strong, balanced muscular framework speeds recovery from injury.
▶ Increases metabolic rate (the rate at which your body burns calories): Strength training adds muscle (or prevents loss of muscle), which has a high-energy requirement. The more muscle you have, the more energy needed for tissue maintenance and the more calories you burn.
▶ Increased bone strength and density: This is important for post-

Learning the lingo

Reps Repetitions of an exercise.
Set The number of reps of an exercise that can be performed to fatigue.
Resistance (load) The amount of weight used in an exercise.
Rest The amount of time of rest in between sets

menopausal women and those prone to osteoporosis and osteoarthritis.
▶ Offsets the loss of muscle that occurs as you age.
▶ Strengthens bones, tendons and ligaments.
▶ Improves physical capacity to perform well at your chosen sport.

Using free weights requires a greater level of skill, coordination and concentration. Though machines have advantages over free weights, such as safety and specificity, they don't teach the body to work as a link system. Instead, they tend to isolate individual muscle groups. Cables, pulleys, dumbbells and barbells are the preferred option for a variety of reasons. Wherever you go in the world, a dumbbell is still a dumbbbell, and the long-term benefits of working out with free weights surpass those of machines.

However, the learning curve for dumbbells and cables (free weights) is a lot greater and so patience, perseverance and proper instruction are the keys to success.

The exercises shown on pages 86–93 aim to integrate and work several muscles simultaneously. You should incorporate them into your workout routine two to three times a week.

Getting started

Technique is everything when it comes to weight/strength training. Quality should be your focus, not quantity. I would much rather a client completed 10 well-executed repetitions than 15–20 poorly executed ones.

Strength training is potentially very dangerous – you can seriously injure yourself if the exercises are not performed properly. Always warm up for 5–10 minutes beforehand or do a set of light weights before you move on to the heavier, more challenging loads.

Form

Bad form will simply lead to injury in the long run, especially for the lower back. Make sure that the only body part that is moving when performing a certain exercise is the one that should be. Learn the proper technique at the start and then concentrate on the exercise, rather than just going through the motions.

Pointers on form Break each movement down into two parts: a lifting phase and a lowering phase. To get the most out of each lift, pause for a second in between the two phases.

Eliminate all unnecessary momentum. Any muscles not involved in the actual exercise should be holding the rest of the body still while the movement is being performed. Your bodyweight should be evenly distributed

Things to remember

► Muscles work in both directions of the movement, so lift and lower the weights in a slow and controlled manner.
► Maintain strict form: Eliminate as much momentum as possible. No bouncing at the bottom of the movement. Each rep should consist of two distinct parts. A down phase, pause; followed by an up phase, pause.
► Make sure to lift to fatigue/failure. This will ensure maximum strength gains. If you stop before you get tired, your gains will be minimised.
► Don't avoid certain exercises; follow a balanced programme.

between both feet further evenly distributed between your heel and the ball of your foot. Repetitions should be slow and controlled.

Building your programme

Follow this protocol for lifting, and you will be on the right track towards a stronger, more efficient running physique.

A strength-training programme can be broken down in to three phases.

1 Preparation: 12–20 reps (beginner).
2 Muscle growth: 8–12 reps (intermediate).
3 Strength and power: 5–8 reps (advanced).

Preparation This phase introduces the body to weight training. Focus on technique and correct form. Time: 4–6 weeks. Recovery between sets: 60 seconds.

Muscle growth Aimed to increase muscle mass. Make sure muscular fatigue is reached between 8–12 reps. It should be the muscle that says stop; and not the brain. Time: 8–12 weeks. Recovery between sets: 60–90 seconds.

Strength and power This is the hardest stage due to the amount of weight you are trying to shift. Time: 4–6 weeks. Recovery between sets: 120+ seconds. The time spent at each phase will depend on your ability.

Exercises for lower body strength

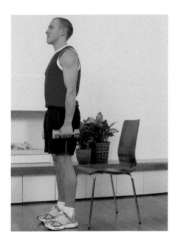 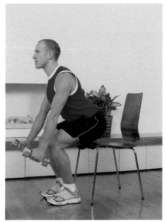 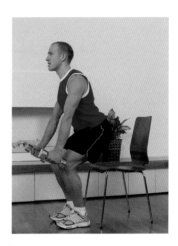

Squat and a half Stand with your feet hip-width apart. Tighten the abdominals and simultaneously flex at the hips and knees as if you were sitting down on the edge of a chair. Lower down to the point where your hips become level with your knees, pause briefly, come halfway back up, lower back down, pause, and then return to full standing position. Keep your eyes looking forward and make sure that your knees stay in line with your toes.

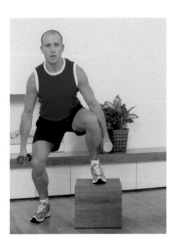 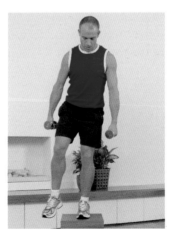

Jump squats Place your right foot on the floor and your left foot on the box, as shown. Push off with your left foot on top of the box and propel yourself over the top of it to the other side. Squat when you land, keeping the right leg on top of the box. Push back over and repeat, squatting each time you land.

One-legged squat Balance on your left foot. If necessary, use the back of a chair to give additional support and balance. Place your right leg out in front of you off the floor. Tighten the abdominals and sit back as if you were sitting on a chair, while maintaining a straight back. Lower down to the point where your thighs are almost parallel to the floor. Repeat on the other side.

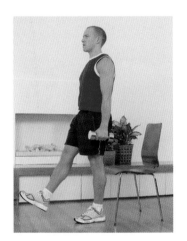

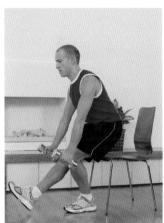

Calf raises Stand on a step with your heels hanging over the edge. Lower your heels down as low as they can go and then stop, so you feel a stretch in your calf muscles. Then push back on to your toes as fast as you can, squeezing the calf muscles as you do so. Alternatives:

▶ One leg at a time.
▶ Holding a weight in one hand.

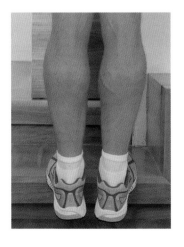

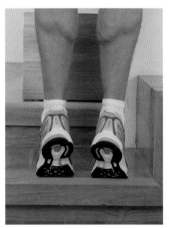

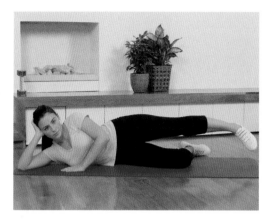 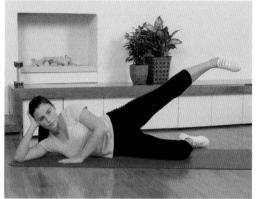

Side-leg raise Lie on your side with your lower leg bent. Lift the upper leg upwards and slightly backwards, and then turn the whole leg in. Then lift the leg slowly 25 times. This strengthens the hip abductors (glutes).

Toe raises Standing tall, keep your heels on the floor and alternately lift your toes up to your shins. Repeat at least 30 times each leg or until the shin muscles start to tire.

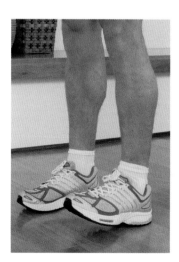 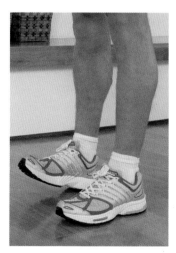

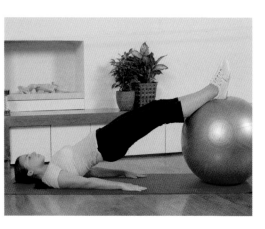 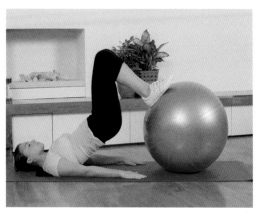

Ball hamstring curls: Lie on the floor on your back and place both feet on top of the ball. Tighten your abdominal muscles and lift your hips off the floor. Then using your heels, pull the ball in towards your bottom, bending your knees. Straighten your legs, while maintaining your hip height and return your back down to the floor.

Heel walk Standing on your heels walk for about 20 paces, turn around, and walk back. Continue until you fatigue the muscles in the front of the shin.

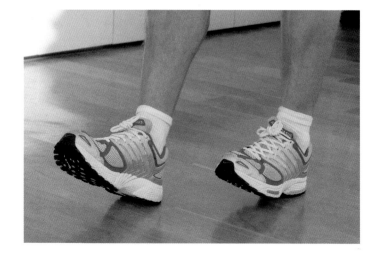

Exercises for upper body strength

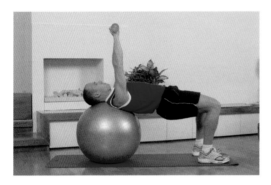

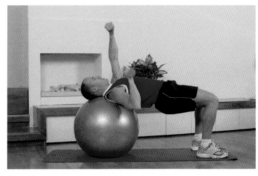

Alternate dumbbell chest press Lying back down on a stability ball, resting your head, neck and shoulders on the ball while maintaining a strong horizontal body position, hold the dumbbells above your chest. Leading with the right elbow lower the dumbbell down to a point level with your chest. As you push the right arm back up, lower the left arm. This exercise will really challenge your balance, so perform it slowly and with extreme care. Keep the breathing as regular as possible.

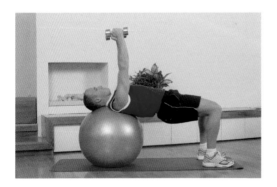

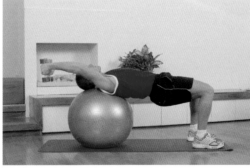

Breathing pullover Lie back down on a stability ball, resting your head, neck and shoulders on the ball. Hold a set of dumbbells with your arms straight above your chest. Bend the elbows slowly and simultaneously lower the dumbbells behind your head. Keeping the elbows bent, pull the dumbbells back over your head and as your upper arms start to become vertical, straighten your arms.

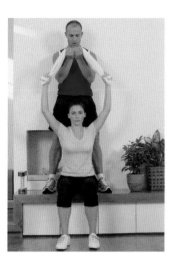

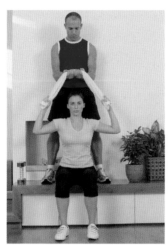

Pull-ups or pulldowns

Pull-ups can be extremely difficult to execute, since you need a lot of upper body strength. Take a fairly wide grip. Breathe out, pulling the shoulderblades together first, then pull the towel down in front of you to a point just below your chin. Always maintain an upright posture, eyes looking straight forward and tension in your core as you perform the pull-down. As an alternative, perform Lat Pulldowns on a machine.

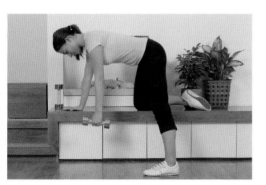

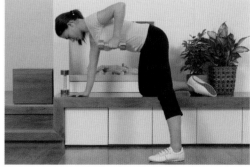

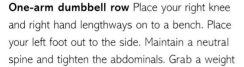

One-arm dumbbell row Place your right knee and right hand lengthways on to a bench. Place your left foot out to the side. Maintain a neutral spine and tighten the abdominals. Grab a weight with the left hand and level the shoulders out. Breathe out and lift the weight up to your side, drawing the elbow close to the body.

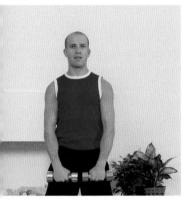 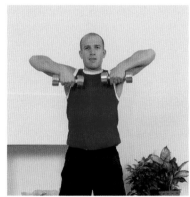 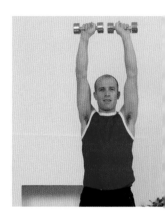

Upright row to shoulder press Hold a set of dumbbells shoulder-width apart at waist level. Leading with the elbows, breathe out and explosively lift the bar to chest level, keeping it close to the body. When the bar reaches chest level, drop and rotate the elbows and catch the bar below your chin. Pause briefly, inhale, exhale and push the bar above your head. Reverse the movement on the way down back down to the start position.

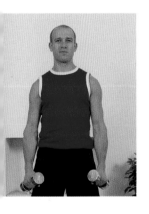 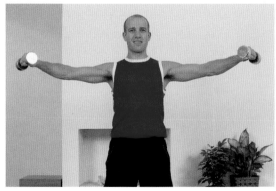 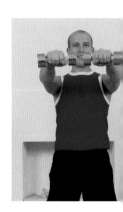

Combination side and front raises Stand with a dumbbell in each hand, feet hip-width apart, knees soft and abdominals engaged. Lift the dumbbells out to the side until shoulder height, then keeping them up, bring them together in front of you. Slowly lower them down to the start position.

Dumbbell curls Holding a dumbbell in each hand, palms facing forwards, keep elbows slightly away from your sides. Lift the dumbbells up towards your shoulders, making sure you don't swing them.

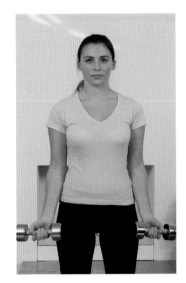 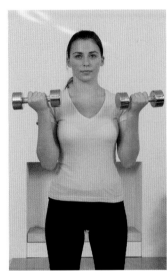

Triceps kickback Bend over to 90 degrees resting your right arm on your right knee. Start with your left arm bent and elbow high. Straighten the arm and pause for a second, squeezing the tricep. Lower the arm slowly, keeping the elbow high. Repeat on the other side.

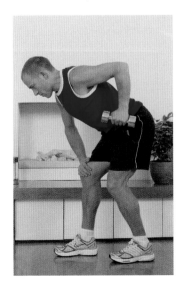 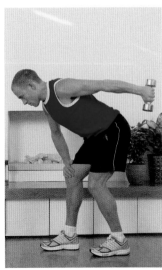

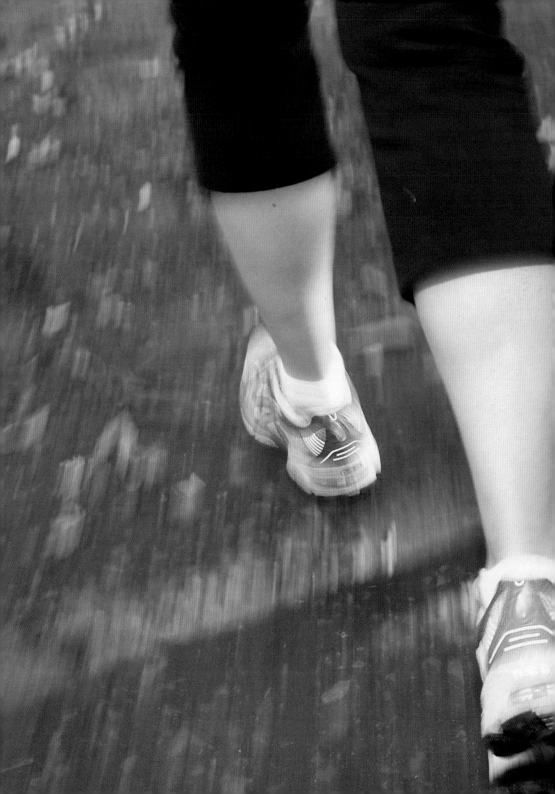

5 Injury & safety

Regular running should help to improve your overall fitness and health, but you should observe some simple measures to avoid illness or injuries. Over-training is a common cause of injury and the key is to listen to your body – allow adequate time between runs to rest and recover properly. If you're running in a gym, always start off gradually and use the treadmill correctly. If you're running outside, do consider the basic safety issues. Try to stick to well-lit streets and busy parks and, if possible, run with a buddy. Always be aware of your surroundings and of other pedestrians and traffic. Run sensibly and safely, and you will minimise the chances of injury and accidents – to yourself and others.

Running and illness

There is no doubt that running places stress on the immune system. During an aerobic workout your body produces free radicals. These free radicals can lead to sickness and disease. But free radicals are not a reason to forego exercise. In fact, your system produces them in response to general environmental exposure. The benefits of running far outweigh any potential free radical damage, and the strengthening of your system through cardiovascular conditioning will actually help your body to withstand negative effects. So at the end of the day, running should improve your general overall health and help prevent colds.

But what to do about the daily run when you feel a cold coming on? If you have a runny or blocked nose, then there's little harm in attempting to run, but be aware of worsening symptoms. If your temperature is increasing and the cold has gone to your chest, give the workout a miss. Concentrate on knocking the symptoms on the head before you start running again. Taking time off can be tough to do, but training when you're not up to it might exacerbate the problem.

Listening to your body

Seasoned athletes will tell you that what one does between training sessions is as important as any time spent on the road or in the gym. Building fitness is a process of adaptation. Your body will require rest, adequate recovery and proper nutrition in order to build muscle and improve systemic (heart and lung) efficiency.

A high number of injuries are caused by over-training. Not letting the body recover sufficiently can put a lot of unnecessary stress on joints and muscles. Rest allows your body to recover, regenerate and adapt. If you are overdoing it, your body will let you know. Headaches, mood swings, pain and fatigue, elevated resting heart rate – all of these symptoms can be caused by over-training. Learning to respect your body's signals is absolutely essential if you are to avoid injury and continue to make progress.

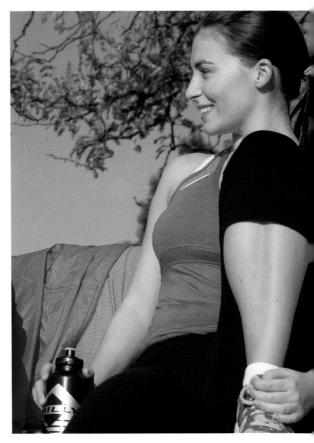

Over-training

Training effectively is all about balance. Smart training means that you know when to challenge your limits and when to rest. For those new to exercise, the 'high' one gets during and after a workout can become intoxicating. The release of endorphins triggers your body's relaxation response, greatly reducing feelings of stress, depression and generalised anxiety. This is one of the benefits of sustained aerobic output, and the motivation for incorporating a workout into your schedule. But it is also the reason that some people become 'hooked', pushing themselves to an extent which is unsustainable and dangerous. For most of us, severe over-training will never be an issue, but if you find yourself compromising other aspects of your life to exercise for increasingly long periods of time, it might be time to step back and assess your programme.

Signs of over-training

If you believe you might be over-training, run through the following checklist. Answering positively to two or more of these questions is a reliable indication that you are venturing into dangerous territory.

- ▶ Does the idea of a day off leave you insecure?
- ▶ Have you cancelled recent social engagements to train instead?
- ▶ Are you more irritable?
- ▶ Are you more fatigued and sleeping fitfully?
- ▶ Do you feel increasingly anxious, distracted and unable to focus?

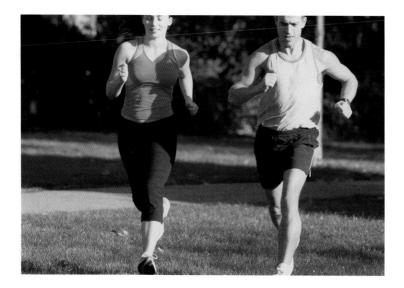

Solutions

. . . .

One way to control an over-training tendency is to exercise with a friend or
a local club. The social element will pull you out of yourself, and help to
counteract obsessiveness. If you are finding it difficult to reduce your training
level, you should arrange to meet with a counsellor or sports psychologist.
They will be able to prescribe effective mechanisms for regulating your over-
training tendency.

Over-training and women

. . . .

One obvious way a woman can determine if she is over-training is by
monitoring her monthly periods. If you find your cycle is becoming irregular,
or if it stops entirely, a condition known as amenorrhoea, then you are
overdoing it. It is very important you regulate your training to a healthy
level as soon as possible, as the long-term effects of amenorrhoea include
loss of bone density (leading to osteoporosis/osteoarthritis) and infertility.

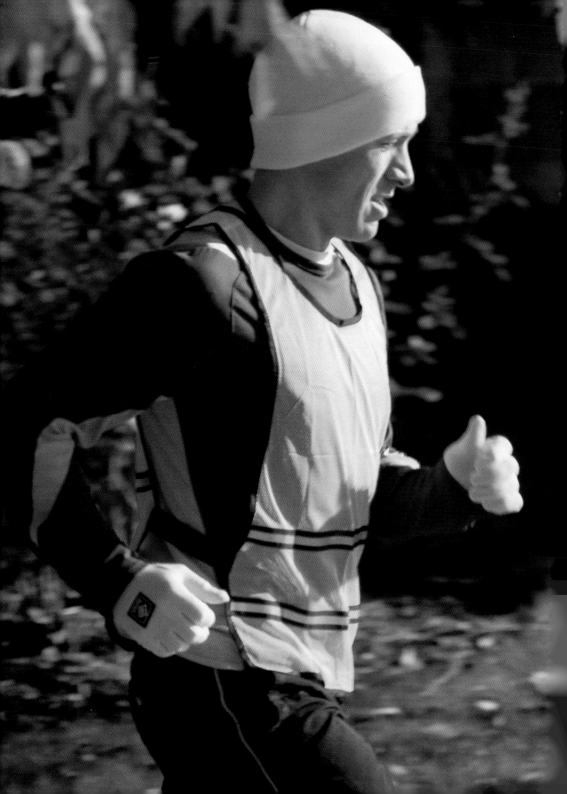

Safety measures

Another issue all runners must contend with, whether in the gym or on the trail, is safety. Many accidents and injuries are the avoidable result of risky decisions, and being aware of the potential pitfalls in your running environment is the best insurance policy. Courtesy while running also plays into the safety category. By observing simple rules of etiquette, you will be forcing yourself to be aware of your surroundings, consequently being ready to adapt in the face of oncoming danger.

On the streets

▶ Do not run in the road. Stick to pavements and parks. This may seem an obvious point, but I cannot tell you the number of times I have come across joggers lazily plodding down the road. Aside from the obvious dangers of oncoming traffic, street-running leaves you susceptible to other traffic dangers like unexpectedly opened car doors. If you must run on the road, make sure you are facing the oncoming traffic.

▶ Look ahead – not down at the ground. If you have the ability to anticipate what might happen, then you can take the necessary steps to avoid an interruption to your run.

▶ Whenever possible, run with a running partner for increased safety.

▶ Carry a mobile phone or some spare change, if possible, in case of an emergency.

▶ Let someone know you are going out for a run.

▶ Avoid wearing headphones, since they reduce awareness of the surrounding environment.

▶ For evening and early morning runners, make sure that you can be seen. Reflective gear is a good way to make oneself more visible.

▶ If you are using reflective straps, then attach them to your ankles or wrists. These body parts move most and hence are most likely to be seen. But remember, although most running gear – shoes, tights, rain jackets – makes use of reflective material, which dramatically improves your visibility for other road and pavement users, you should still exercise caution, especially when running in urban areas.

▶ Run on well-lit roads and in well-lit and busy parks. If you can't see the ground directly in front of you, then it is time to seek out an alternative.

▶ Women running out of doors should also take a few extra precautions: carry a personal alarm if you are in an urban environment, stay away from dark areas, don't wear any jewellery and try to vary your routine as much as possible.

Etiquette

▶ Being aware of road users and other pedestrians is a big part of running outdoors.

▶ Try to be aware of what is going on around you, especially in built-up areas or crowded locations. Keep your vision as open as possible.

▶ When running around blind corners, take them wide to avoid unnecessary collisions. Obviously a collision is frightening for someone who is not expecting a runner to come around the corner full pelt. There is nothing worse than running straight into an unsuspecting person.

▶ Don't expect pedestrians to get out of your way; always choose the path of least resistance. Give people a wide berth – you never know when they're going to stop dead in their tracks or change direction suddenly.

▶ Try to visualise the worst-case scenario and imagine how you would respond, then the appropriate action can be taken to avoid accidents.

▶ Always assume that motorists have not seen you. Making eye contact with the driver ensures that they know you are there. If a driver does let you cross, it's always polite to thank them with a nod or a wave.

▶ So, be aware while running. Keep vigilant. Dogs, kids, the elderly, tourists, kerbs, hidden driveways, people exiting shops, cyclists, people pointing or changing direction suddenly are all potential pitfalls, and can turn a relaxing workout into a trip to hospital. Staying alert means that you'll have many more fitness building runs in the future!

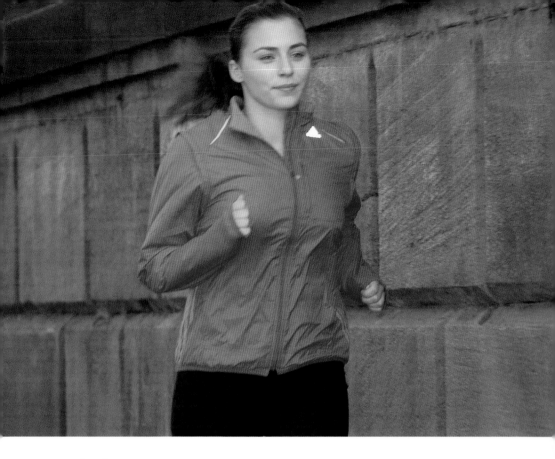

In the gym

- ▶ Do not hold on to the side rails of the treadmill while running. Not only do you look ridiculous, but it is dangerous. Slow your pace to a level you can maintain while letting your arms move freely.
- ▶ Don't crank the treadmill up to running pace before climbing aboard. It might sound obvious, but in fact it is a common error in first-time treadmill runners.
- ▶ If it is your first time on the equipment, start off with a walk, gradually increasing your pace as you feel more comfortable.
- ▶ Unless it is an emergency, do not go from a full run to a complete stop. Decrease you speed slowly to prevent injury or damage to the equipment.
- ▶ Don't jump off while the machine is moving.

Common running injuries and their causes

At some point in your running career it will happen you'll suffer from some sort of injury – it just goes with the territory. However, by listening to your body's early on you can prevent lasting damage and knowing how to deal with the problem will get you back on your feet as quickly as possible.

The main cause of injuries amongst beginners is that there is a tendency to do too much to soon. Being keen is good and, as a trainer, it is great to see, but sometimes being too keen can get you into trouble and lead to injury. Some other common injury-inducing factors are:

▶ Inappropriate footwear.
▶ Previous injury.
▶ Not listening to your body. Don't ignore pain. It's your body's way of trying to tell you something.

Common running injuries

Hip: Piriformis syndrome
Feeling Dull ache in the butt, often accompanied by pain in the sciatic nerve.
Cause Wear and tear of shoes, running on cambered surfaces and pelvis misalignment.
Fix Rolling on a tennis ball will massage the affected area, new shoes and running on softer surfaces.

Hamstrings
Feeling Searing pain, dull ache.
Cause Not warming up properly/weak muscle.
Fix RICED treatment (see page 107), strength and stretch.

Runner's knee
Feeling Pain under or to the side of the knee cap.
Cause Overpronation, inappropriate running shoes or excessive training. Knee pain in runners is quite common and can come from poor muscle balance round the hip and knee.
Fix Strengthen weak muscles, wear the shoe for your foot type and reduce training.

Achilles tendon
Feeling Tightness/inflexibility/soreness.
Cause Incorrect or worn out running shoes, excessively tight calves, overpronation, wearing high heels and over training.
FIX: RICED treatment, lower and upper calf stretches, fitting of correct running shoes, reducing training volume.

Plantar fasciitis
Feeling Pain and tenderness from heel to mid-sole.
Cause Usually caused by overpronation or poor flexibility in the calves, Achilles and hamstrings.
Fix Stretch and strengthen Achilles and calf. Roll your foot over a tennis ball to keep the ligaments loose. Reduce inflammation with ice.

Chafing
Feeling Pain and discomfort in your armpits and between your inner thighs.
Cause Friction from the running motion.
Fix Apply Vaseline to the affected areas. Avoid wearing vests. Wea longer shorts such as cycling shorts.

Shin splints
Feeling The name is slang for what is officially called 'Medial Tibial Stress Syndrome', and can be identified by a pain down the front or inside part of the lower leg. The symptoms include aching, throbbing or tenderness down the shin. The pain is usually quite mild at first but with continued training can worsen quickly and become very uncomfortable.

Cause Shin splints occur due to impact with the ground. Muscles become weak and short and unable to do the job they were designed for. It affects people with flat feet or over pronators as well as those that run on hard surfaces with inadequate cushioning. Beginners also suffer especially due to doing too much too soon.

Fix Buying the right footwear and vary running surfaces and avoid hill. To avoid losing fitness cross train. Stretching can help.

Stomach cramps

Feeling Dodgy stomach, bloating, and nausea or even mid-run diarrhoea are common amongst a great number of runners.

Cause There is no single cause for these ailments, but a combination of the wrong food choices, slight dehydration, reduced blood flow to the stomach and lower intestines, and the bouncing action of running, can turn even the strongest stomach into a cement mixer. Certain things are know to get your stomachs upset include too much food, the sugar found in fizzy drinks and the butterflies you get before a race.

Modify your pre-run nutrition. It can take a while to find the optimal nutritional balance for your best performance. A combination of trial and error will enable you to distinguish: what foods you can eat before you train, how much you need to eat and how long you need to digest.

Blisters

Feeling Extreme discomfort on the skin surface where the blister is located.

Cause Blisters occur due to friction causing layers of skin to pull apart and the space created between them to fill up with liquid.

Fix Some say leave them alone and let them heal however others believe they should be burst and treated. To burst a blister, sterilise a needle and make a small incision into the blister allowing the fluid to drain. Let the blister breath and then place a plaster/dressing over it. To keep blisters at bay, correctly fitted footwear is a must.

So what do you do? Go straight to the physio? Ignore it? The first thing you should do is to make a note in your training diary recording the date of onset and the pain's intensity. If you don't keep track of the injury, before long it will be a lot worse, lingering for months. If you haven't kept a record, you will convince yourself it's improving, when it may actually be worsening.

The second thing you should do is to consult a physiotherapist and listen to their advice. Too many of us assume we know the best solution for our own bodies, and attempt to fix problems beyond our capabilities. Self-diagnosis is difficult unless it's a previous injury that has reoccurred. Typically injuries arise from doing too much too soon, or increasing distances, times, or intensities too sharply.

Self-treatment of potential injuries

If the injury is relatively simple or you are familiar with the problem from previous experience, you may be able to forego the physio and solve the problem yourself. The basic steps to treatment are:

▶ Ice the injured area for 10-minute periods 3-4 times a day.
▶ Take an anti-inflammatory to reduce pain and inflammation.
▶ Cut back on your training, and if necessary, rest up for a few days.
▶ Stretch the area with care.
▶ Don't try and run through an injury, it's likely to make it a lot worse.

RICED

Every athlete is well acquainted with the RICE system for treating injury. By running through these steps consistently, you should be able to solve most minor problems. However, if after a few days the pain has not subsided or has gotten worse, then consult a specialist as soon as possible.

▶ **R**est: minimise use of the injusred area.
▶ **I**ce: 10-15 minutes 3-4 x a day.
▶ **C**ompression: Wrap the area.
▶ **E**levation: lift the affected area above your heart while resting.
▶ **D**iagnosis: seek professional help.

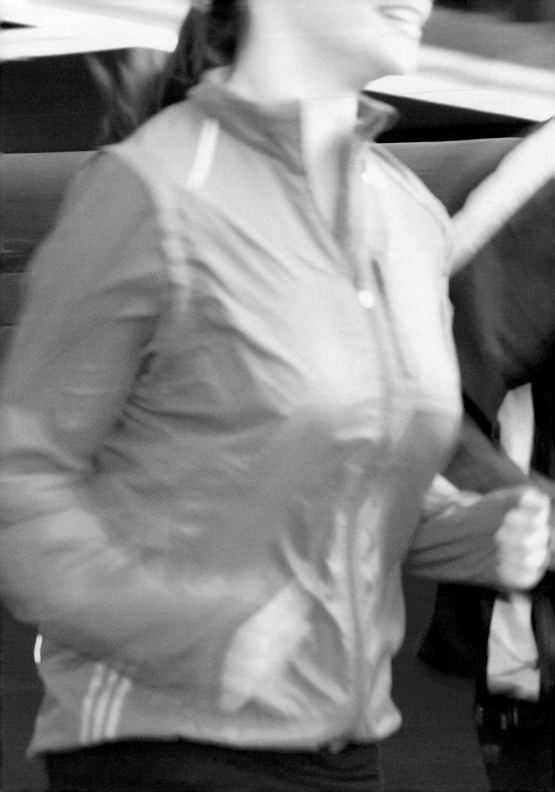

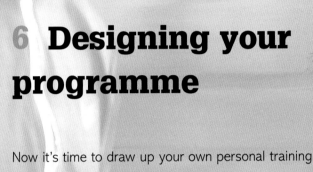

6 Designing your programme

Now it's time to draw up your own personal training programme, based on your goals – do you want to get fit, lose weight or actively compete? It's important to choose a running environment that is convenient for you, so that you will keep running regularly. To get the most out of the running experience, it's a good idea to vary your routine at least once a week, so that you do some more challenging runs. You can also incorporate other activities such as swimming, cycling or weight training. There are useful ways to motivate and monitor yourself like joining a running club or entering a race.

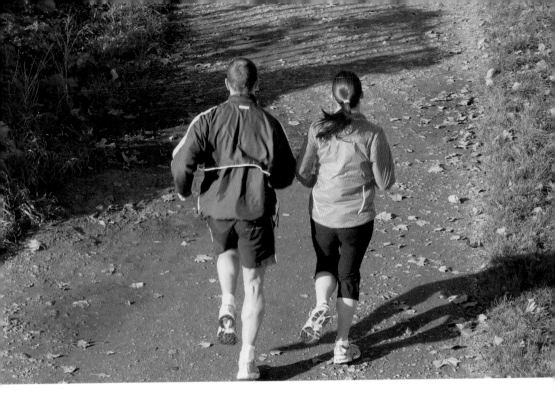

Setting your goals

If you've read this far, then you now have a solid foundation of information about running and exercise in general. You understand that becoming fit is about achieving balance in your training and nutrition. You are familiar with the potential pitfalls, the injuries and safety risks to watch for, and hopefully you have begun to apply these principles to visualising your own programme. In this chapter, I will help you through the basics of designing a sustainable and effective training regimen. We will explore the impact different sorts of goals have on your plans, and review the techniques for creating a programme to suit you.

Why set goals?

To get the most out of your running, it is important you set clear, realistic and attainable goals. Are you striving to participate in competition? Hoping to lose excess weight? Or perhaps you simply want to build a healthier lifestyle, deriving all the available benefits? Identifying where you want to go makes it possible to map the route. If you don't have a clearly defined sense of what you are aiming for, it will be difficult to find the motivation to maintain your programme.

Important considerations

- ▶ Make the goal realistic. Is it possible? Can you do it? Something that is a little out of your comfort zone would be ideal. Saying that, it may be that simply running is a challenge, and sticking to your basic workout is tough enough! Listen to your body, but push yourself at the same time.
- ▶ Make the goal specific. Can you measure it? Distance and time are easy ways to set benchmarks and probably the most popular options. Stay away from the temptation to track progress through your weight. It is not an accurate measure of fitness, as weight fluctuates superficially all the time, and you may lose motivation when the numbers don't meet your expectations.
- ▶ Get someone else involved or tell others about your new goals. Having a cheering section will place you under a little bit of pressure, which can only be a good thing.
- ▶ Commit to a charity or event – something that will keep you training for the big day.
- ▶ Write the goal down on your calendar or in big letters in your diary. Or make a sign for the fridge – this is a great way to stay motivated and keep yourself on the right nutritional track!
- ▶ And never forget: reward yourself! Pick a unique way to celebrate your accomplishment when you reach your goal. Having a prize at the end of the rainbow is another great motivator.

Choosing your running environment

One of the most important factors determining training success is consistency. Choosing a comfortable and convenient option is essential if you are to stick with it. For some, the gym is impractical; for others it is the only option. Many health clubs have crèche facilities these days and so if you are trying to balance training with childcare, this can be particularly convenient.

Training outside

To accelerate your progress, I believe that combining a variety of environments is key. Running outside promotes a number of fitness elements, which running indoors does not. Changes in terrain require increased muscular development and agility. The ever-changing environment and landscape keep you alert and aware, improving your concentration and focus.

Training in the gym

Running in a gym or at home does have its advantages. Primarily, training inside is not weather dependent, you need less gear and the social aspect of a gym environment can be added motivation to stick with it. Additionally, if you are running on a treadmill it is easier to keep a consistent pace, something very important for beginners looking to build a stable running foundation. Lastly, working out in the gym means you will be able to cross-train more effectively, as there are numerous types of machines and resistance training facilities. This keeps it interesting and balancing the different modalities will also accelerate your progress and prevent injury.

Training at home

Many exercisers find running on a treadmill easier than road running. This could be due to the lack of wind resistance, smooth ground surface, single direction or the fact that you can zone out on a treadmill. If you do buy one, make sure that you still get outside at least once or twice a week.

Treadmills

If you are going to buy a treadmill, then there are several things you need to bear in mind:

► How much space do you have? If space is an issue, there are many models on the market that fold away.
► How much can you afford? The commercial treadmills within gyms are bigger and sturdier than the home versions. Shop around and have a go on different models. Generally speaking, the more you are willing to spend, the higher the quality of the equipment. Buy a cheap treadmill and it will feel like running on a cheap treadmill. Before long, you won't be using it and will be back using the ones in the gym or worse yet, not running at all.
► Is the top speed fast enough?
► Does it have a gradient setting on it?
► Is it user friendly? Is it easy to operate?
► If you cannot complement your indoor running with the occasional outdoor run, you should make certain your treadmill has a variety of programmes.
► Where are you going to put the treadmill? You don't really want to be facing the wall when you're running. Placing it near a window or entertainment centre will make the exercise more enjoyable.
► Does your room have good ventilation?
► Does the treadmill come with a good warranty?

Types of goals

Depending on your aims, specific training programmes should be followed. It is important to target your programme to meet your priorities: weight loss, cardiovascular health and competition. Let's review some of the basic training protocols behind each one:

Running for weight loss

For many people, weight loss and weight management are primary concerns. Recent behavioural studies have linked everything from success in the workplace to finding love, with our pant sizes, so for most of us a concern with the numbers on the scale is almost inevitable.

Running for weight loss requires some specific measures. Nutrition is key, and as I tell my clients, if you start running without modifying your diet, you are not going to see the progress you desire. Your runs should be long sessions at a lowered intensity – well within the aerobic zone. Moderate intensity exercise is the optimal conditioning framework for sustained weight loss. You should try to run in the mornings, before breakfast, as this forces your body to utilise fat stores for energy, rather than the energy of the day's fuel intake.

Running for cardiovascular (CV) conditioning

If it is your general health you are seeking to improve, designing your programme to improve cardiovascular function is a good approach. The main differences between a routine specified to accelerate fat loss and a routine targeting cardio improvement are the variations in intensity and length of the exercise sessions. CV training requires you to push your heart rate into the Lactate Threshold and Max VO2 zones, forcing the body's system to adapt.

The key to successful CV training is to place your body under just enough stress so that it is forced to improve.

Weight loss checklist

▶ Be persistent and consistent: you need to commit to a full schedule of training days. Once or twice a week is not going to cut it if weight loss is your aim. You should try to exercise at least five times a week, and complement your non-running days with a bit of cross-training such as swimming or cycling. Basically, aim to do some form of exercise every day. And remember, every exercise session is variable, it doesn't have to last an hour each time – feel free to split it up as your schedule permits. Some days you might only have the time for a 15-minute power walk. The most important thing is that you do something.

▶ On the days that you're running/training, cut down on the volume of food that you're eating. Eating too much will lead to stomach cramps and side stitches. Also, many people feel that running gives them a license to eat more than they normally would, or to allow themselves foods they would generally avoid. Do not make this mistake. Going out running does not mean you can store calorie credits to spend on your favourite foods.

▶ Food/nutrition is the key: running alone won't help you lose weight. Though it will improve internal fitness, the wrong food choices will leave you heavy. In fact, I like to tell my clients that real weight management/loss is determined by nutritional choices. Eat 'lean and clean' food, i.e. unprocessed, fresh and lower on the Glycemic Index (see page 41). By opting for these lowered GI foods, you keep sugar levels stable and your food cravings at bay.

▶ Set yourself small goals. I explained that measuring progress by the scales wasn't always a bright idea. Weight is unstable and the slightest change in hydration levels or internal processes can register on the scales. With my clients, I use girth measurements (hips, waist, thighs) instead. This way, we can track real progress – I also have them establish a 6-week and a 12-week target. This helps to keep the motivation levels high.

▶ Keep a food diary. This is the best way to monitor your nutrition and stay on track. Writing down what you eat and when can be very surprising. Many people find they are taking in far more than they had thought. By recording your intake, you will be able to identify negative patterns that might be hindering your progress.

The recognised training threshold for developing cardiovascula/aerobic fitness is 20–60 minutes at 60–85 per cent of your Working Heart Rate (WHR). Depending on your fitness level and the type of session selected, your target HR will fall anywhere along this scale. As your body adapts, you will be able to enjoy longer, more intense workouts while remaining within the same HR zone. By monitoring your Heart Rate levels, you can ensure that you continue to train effectively as this adaptation occurs. Here are some quick pointers to optimise your cardio workouts:

▶ Use the equations for calculating your different HR zones in Chapter 1 to determine your Lactate Threshold and Max VO2 zones. This will provide you with a foundation around which you can structure your training programme.

▶ Vary your runs by including interval-training sessions. By pushing your HR into one of the more taxing zones and interspersing the harder intensities with recovery intensities, you will your fitness programme safely and effectively.

▶ For Lactate Threshold conditioning (about 80–90 per cent of your maximum) try the following plan: use an interval training system. Get into your Lactate Threshold zone for 5–10+ minutes and then reduce your pace to bring your heart rate back down, and recover for an equal amount of time. Repeat the cycle three times. These intense efforts will get the body used to functioning with greater amounts of lactate build-up, thereby improving your cardiovascular fitness.

▶ For Max VO2 conditioning (90–100 per cent of your maximum) follow this model: by far the hardest and most uncomfortable training zone, your Max VO2 puts your heart rate to its highest level. This requires great effort, but a few minutes once a week will pay huge dividends over time, especially improving your overall strength and power. As with Lactate Threshold intervals, these brief bursts of effort can be incorporated between aerobic zone intervals. Warm up in your aerobic zone for 10 minutes, then do 3–10 repeats of 1–3 minutes at a hard pace alternated with an easy recovery for 1–3 minutes. Follow this with 10–20 minutes of cool-down in your aerobic zone.

▶ For the running novice, cardiovascular conditioning is a great idea, but must be done carefully. I advise at least 4–6 weeks of conditioning training within the aerobic zone to build a solid aerobic foundation before attempting to include more challenging zones into your training schedule.

Running for competitions

You might have started to run for other reasons, but once you have achieved a basic level of fitness, entering a race or fun run can be a good way to step up to the next level. Races and fun runs are great motivators. Having an event to train for puts you under a bit of pressure, which is a good thing. It requires you to train with increased direction, focus and commitment.

I have coached a number of my clients to prepare for running competitions. From marathons to simple 5 km (3 mile) fun runs, the secret to proper race training is building time and speed in a methodical, well-planned fashion.

Interval training, long-distance runs, incorporating resistance training – all these components are important for the competitor in training.

Competitive running checklist

▶ Vary your runs. Alternate your aims on different days: one day run for speed; the next day run for distance. Below is a guide to the different sorts of training runs one can do.

▶ Run with a club or friend. Training with others will push you and acclimate you to the feeling of competition.

▶ Get in the gym and hit the weights. To build your speed and endurance for racing you will need to complement your running training with other forms of exercise.

▶ Follow a well-balanced nutritional plan. Test-drive your pre-competition meal by mimicking race day conditions a few times before the actual event.

The importance of variety

In order to enjoy the running experience, you have to aim for variety in your training. Even if you only change the routine once a week, it just puts a different spin on things. It can rekindle your interest and enthusiasm, especially when you don't feel particularly motivated.

If you are finding it hard to come up with new ideas for training, remember you can always run your favourite routes in reverse. Joining a running club or group is another great way to spice up your training programme. Running clubs do cater for all abilities so don't be put off by the worry that you have to be fit to join a club.

Change the route you run on a regular basis. Boredom can set in quite easily if you run the same route time after time. Find a local map and plot new routes. It won't take you long to come up with several runs that give you a lot of variety and scope.

You will find that your fitness improves more rapidly with the incorporation of variety. To measure your progress, have one run that you use as your 'control run'. This is the run you do once or twice a month to set a new personal best. Call it your very own personal fitness test.

Types of runs

Long Slow Distance runs (LSD)

These are runs that you gradually build towards with your shorter workouts. The idea is to add a little more time each time you run. When you feel ready to meet the challenge, pick a day where you have enough time to enjoy the experience. Long runs are a great way to improve your general fitness, as the sustained exercise will boost your oxygen uptake within the muscles. Pacing yourself is key for these, as you don't want to set off too quickly and burn yourself out. Here are some good tips for designing your long runs:

LSD tips

▶ Heart rates for this type of training are around 60–75 per cent of MHR.

▶ Add no more than 5–10 minutes (10 per cent) to your long runs on a weekly basis.

▶ By having a longer run at the weekend you will significantly increase your stamina. Weekends tend to be the ideal time for these longer runs because you usually have more time, but there is no reason why your long run can't be done during the week if that is easier.

The Fartlek

This is Swedish term that literally means 'speed play'. It involves changing speed over a variety of distances and with a variable recovery. A good place to try a Fartlek, if you are new to the technique, is a local school track. Most tracks have distance markers to help you manage your interval lengths. Speed work makes you a faster runner.

Ongoing maintenance

Over the course of three weeks, build up your mileage, then on the 4th week reduce it by 30–35 per cent.

For weeks 5, 6 and 7, build mileage again, and cut back in week 8 by 30–35 per cent.

▶ One week every month, reduce your training by a third.

▶ Take regular rest days – these involve not running at all.

▶ Don't push yourself all the time, mix up the intensity of your running.

▶ Don't feel guilty about taking a couple of days off.

The easy run

There is really only one rule of thumb here – on an easy run make sure you take it easy! Aim to get in an easy run once a week. This will keep you from burning out and reduce your risk of injury.

Tempo runs

These are tough workouts, but the benefits are huge, especially for your overall fitness level. A tempo run should feel comfortably hard, with the emphasis on 'hard'. It is meant to be difficult. Some people will shy away from this type of training because it is too uncomfortable. You're running in your Lactate Threshold zone, roughly 80–90 per cent of your WHR.

The benefit of this type of training is that it conditions the body to cope with the build-up of lactic acid. The body is constantly producing lactic acid, but when you're working aerobically, the body is able to rid itself of the lactate as quickly as it's produced. However, at higher heart rates, when the body is working anaerobically (without oxygen) lactate is generated at such great rates that the body can't neutralise it quickly enough. Consequently, it accumulates. Conditioning your body to tolerate varying levels of lactic acid build-up is an important part of increasing your fitness level.

Hill runs

If you would like to see your fitness level go through the roof, then add some hills into your route. Obviously, the steeper the hill, the greater the effort; but the greater the effort, the better the long-term results. Running hills increases calorie burn, as well as boosting your aerobic and anaerobic systems.

Hill Running technique Drive hard with the legs and really make use of your arms when running uphill. Maintain your momentum over the top of the hill. A wide variety of muscles are used when running up hills. More muscle fibres are recruited due to the effort needed to get to the top.

For beginners, aim to run at a lower gradient, a slower speed and for shorter distances. Start with one or two hills, building up slowly to 10. As your confidence grows along with your fitness, find a steeper, longer hill and run faster.

Off-road

There are far too many treadmill runners around, and not enough people willing to venture outside into the elements. There is no better feeling than running in the fresh air through a wood, jumping over branches, dodging puddles and rocks, and constantly changing direction. The trail surface is normally a lot softer as well, so some cross-country running will help to reduce stress on your joints while strengthening them. If you are after a great workout that will improve your agility, balance, core strength and sense of adventure, find a trail.

Running alternatives

Don't forget that a truly successful running programme will also incorporate other forms of exercise. Activities like swimming, cycling and elliptical training are all excellent options for increasing your fitness and engaging muscle groups in new ways. Obviously, weight training (see page 82) is an important complement to any programme, and I strongly believe you need to include a basic resistance programme in your training regimen.

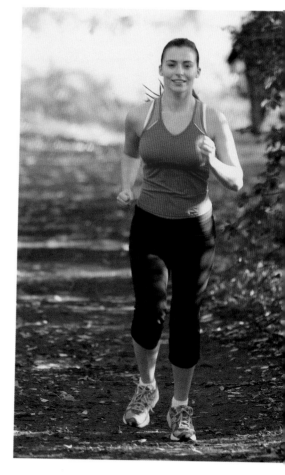

Running programmes

Getting started on a running programme can be extremely daunting for a lot of people. You should ease into a programme by combining walking and running. A beginner can be quickly turned off running simply because they start to fast or try to run too far or for too long. There is nothing worse than feeling like your lungs are going to explode on your first outing.

There is no reason why you can't be transformed from a couch potato to 30 minute runner in 8 weeks. The only requirement is that you be consistent and follow the programme.

Guidelines for a run/walk programme

▶ Take at least a day off in between each run.
▶ Runs can be done inside or outside.
▶ Try to pick a route outside that is relatively flat.
▶ Use the walk as a recovery.
▶ The run pace should be steady, you should be able hold a conversation.
▶ It's ok to repeat a week or go back a week.
▶ Stick to the plan, please avoid advancing to quickly.

Guidelines for a half marathon programme

▶ The programme on page 125 assumes that you are already running two or three miles at a time, three or four times a week.
▶ By the later stages of the programme, you should know how your body is coping with the training load. If 22 miles a week is hard work, try cutting down week 9 to 15 miles in total.
▶ In the final week, you'll be tapering; by reducing the amount of running, you'll build up extra energy stores in your legs ready for the race.
▶ You can arrange the training days as you like, but try to have a rest day after a hard day.

Walk/run programme (8 weeks)

		Run	Walk	Times	Total time
Week 1	Session 1	1 min	4 min	X 4	20 mins
	Session 2	1 min	4 min	X 5	25 mins
	Session 3	2 min	3 min	X 4	20 min
Week 2	Session 1	2 min	3 min	X 5	25 mins
	Session 2	2.5 min	2.5 min	X 5	25 mins
	Session 3	3 min	2 min	X 5	25 min
Week 3	Session 1	3 min	2 min	X 6	30 mins
	Session 2	3.5 min	1.5 min	X 5	25 mins
	Session 3	4 min	1 min	X 5	25 min
Week 4	Session 1	4 min	1 min	X 6	30 mins
	Session 2	6 min	2 min	X 4	32 mins
	Session 3	6 min	1 min	X 4	28 min
Week 5	Session 1	8 min	2 min	X 2	20 mins
	Session 2	8 min	1 min	X 2	27 mins
	Session 3	10 min	2 min	X 2	24 min
Week 6	Session 1	10 min	1 min	X 3	33 mins
	Session 2	12 min	2 min	X 2	28 mins
	Session 3	12 min	1 min	X 2	26 min
Week 7	Session 1	15 min	2 min	X 2	34 mins
	Session 2	15 min	1 min	X 2	32 mins
	Session 3	18 min	2 min	X 2	40 min
Week 8	Session 1	20 min	2 min	X 1	22 mins
	Session 2	20 min	1 min	X 2	42 mins
	Session 3	30 min	0 min	X 1	30 min

10 k/6 miles (8 weeks)

	Session 1	Session 2	Session 3
Week 1	3 km/2 miles easy, then 4 x 400m fast, with 3-min jog recoveries, then 3 km/2 miles easy	4 km/2.5 miles easy, 3 km/2 miles fast, jog to cool down	4 km/ 2.5 miles easy
Week 2	3 km/2 miles easy, then 4 x 600m or 2 mins fast, with 3-min jog recoveries, then 3 km/2 miles easy	15 mins easy, 15 mins fast but controlled, jog to finish	5.5 km/ 3–4 miles easy
Week 3	4 km/2.5 miles easy, then 4 x 800m or 3 mins fast, with 3-min jog recoveries, then 3 km/2 miles easy	30–40 mins relaxed, including some hills	8 km/ 5 miles easy
Week 4	3 km/2 miles easy, then 8 x 400m or 70–80 seconds fast, with 3-min jog recoveries, then 3 km/2 miles easy	8 km/5 miles, first half at about 70% effort, second half at about 85% effort	9 km/ 5–6 miles easy
Week 5	3 km/2 miles easy, then 8 x 500m or 90–100 seconds fast, with 3-min jog recoveries, then 3 km/2 miles easy	35–45 mins fartlek with varied efforts and recoveries	10.5 km/ 6–7 miles easy
Week 6	4 km/2.5 miles easy, then 5 x 800m or 3 mins fast, with 3-min jog recoveries, then 4 km/2.5 miles easy	10.5 km/6–7 miles, gradual acceleration in 4 km/2.5 mile segments	12 km/ 7.5 miles easy
Week 7	5 km/3 miles easy, then 10 x 400m or 70–80 seconds fast, with 3-min jog recoveries, then 5 km/3 miles easy	Warm up, then 4 x 1.5 km/1 mile or 6 mins fast, with 3-min jog recoveries, then cool down	13 km/ 8 miles easy
Week 8	5 km/3 miles easy, then 5–6 x 500m or 90–100 seconds fast, with 3-min jog recoveries, then 5 km/3 miles easy	7 km/4–5 miles easy	Race

SCHEDULE BY SEAN FISHPOOL AND BUD BALDARO

Half marathon//20.5 km (10 weeks)

Week	Session 1	Session 2	Session 3	Session 4
1	6.5 km/ 4 miles slow	5 km/ 3 miles slow	6.5 km/ 4 miles easy	5 km/ 3 miles timed
2	5 km/ 3 miles easy	5 km/3 miles, with 50m bursts	5 km/ 3 miles easy	8–9 km/ 5–6 miles slow
3	6.5 km/ 4 miles easy	6.5 km/4 miles, with 100m bursts	5 km/3 miles, timed, plus slow 1.5 km/1 mile slow	12 km/7.5 miles (or one hour)
4	6.5 km/ 4 miles easy	6.5 km/4 miles, with 30-second bursts	6.5 km/ 4 miles easy	12–13 km/8 miles slow (or one hour)
5	6.5 km/4 miles (or 35–40 mins) easy, off-road	7 km/4–5 miles of fast and slow, with bursts up hills	6.5 km/4 miles (or 35–40 mins) easy, off-road	15 km/9–10 miles steady, or a 10 km/ 6 mile race
6	5.5 km/ 3–4 miles easy	1.5 km/1 mile jog, then 2 x 5 mins fast, with 5-min slow jog recovery	6.5 km/ 4 miles easy	15 km/ 9–10 miles slow
7	5.5 km/ 3–4 miles easy, off-road if possible	3 miles with faster bursts	3 miles easy	Warm up, then 10 km/6 mile race, then 10 mins walking or jogging
8	7 km/ 4–5 miles easy	1.5 km/1 mile jog, then 2 x 7–8 mins fast, with 5-min jog recoveries	6.5 km/4 miles on grass, with fast bursts	18.5 km/ 11–12 miles, as slow as you like
9	5.5 km/3–4 miles easy, on soft ground	1.5 km/1 mile jog, then 2 x 5 mins fast, with 5-min slow jog recoveries	6.5 km/4 miles easy on grass	15 km/ 9–10 miles slow
10	5 km/3 miles easy, off-road	1.5 km/1 mile jog, then 1.5 km/1 mile at race speed, then 1.5 km/1 mile jog	3 km/2 mile jog	Race day

SCHEDULE BY SEAN FISHPOOL AND BUD BALDARO

Index